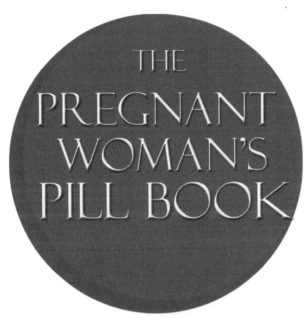

THE PREGNANT WOMAN'S PILL BOOK

A Guide to the Most Frequently Used Over-the-Counter Medications

THEODORE M. PECK, M.D.

Frederick Fell
Publishers, Inc.
Since 1945

Frederick Fell Publishers, Inc.
2131 Hollywood Blvd., Suite 305, Hollywood, FL 33020
Phone: (954) 925-5242   Fax: (954) 925-5244
Web Site: www.FellPub.com

Frederick Fell Publishers, Inc.

2131 Hollywood Boulevard, Suite 305

Hollywood, Florida 33020

954-925-5242

e-mail: fellpub@aol.com

Visit our Web site at www.fellpub.com

This publication is designed to provide accurate and authoritative information in regard to the subject matter covered. It is sold with the understanding that the publisher is not engaged in rendering legal, accounting, or other professional service. If legal advice or other assistance is required, the services of a competent professional person should be sought. From A Declaration of Principles jointly adopted by a Committee of the American Bar Association and a Committee of Publishers.

The information in this book is not intended as medical advice. Its intention is solely informational and educational. It is assumed that the reader will consult a medical or health professional should the need for one be warranted.

Library of Congress Cataloging-in-Publication Data

Peck, Theodore M.

The pregnant woman's pill book : a guide to the most frequently used over-the-counter medications / by Theodore M. Peck.

p. cm.

Includes bibliographical references and index.

ISBN 0-88391-102-7 (pbk. : alk. paper)

1. Reproductive toxicology. 2. Pregnancy. 3. Drugs,

Nonprescription--Toxicology. 4. Reproduction--Effect of drugs on. I.

Title.

RA1224.2.P43 2003

616.6'5071--dc22

2003014765

10 9 8 7 6 5 4 3 2 1

Graphic Design: Elena Solis

THE PREGNANT WOMAN'S PILL BOOK

A Guide to the Most Frequently Used Over-the-Counter Medications

THEODORE M. PECK, M.D.

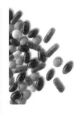

Acknowledgments

This book could not have been made without a great deal of help, graciously provided by three terrific women. The bulk of the typing and secretarial work was ably provided by Jessie Reinhart, who, herself, was pregnant much of the time this book was being written. The accuracy of the information was double-checked by Janet L. Williams MS, C.G.C., who has provided excellent genetic counseling and teratologic services for many years to pregnant women at the Gundersen Clinic in La Crosse, Wisconsin. Additional support and proof-reading was lovingly provided by my wife, Vicki, who has been a great inspiration for my brief writing career and has co-authored our other book, Empowered Pregnancy.

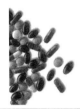

Dedication

This book is dedicated to all those pregnant women who have suffered unnecessarily in the past because of fear of using over-the-counter medications. It is my fervent hope that the information in this book will be helpful in reducing the many annoying aggravations of an otherwise wonderful, amazing, and fascinating time.

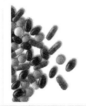

TABLE OF CONTENTS

Chapter One

General Information

Nearly every American adult has experienced minor health problems which have been relieved, partially or completely, by taking non-prescription, or over-the-counter (OTC) drugs. These problems include such everyday ailments as headaches, muscle or joint pains, cold symptoms, allergies, diarrhea, and constipation, just to name a few.

These and similar health problems may not be serious enough to seek medical attention, and yet are disturbing enough to affect work productivity, school work and attendance, personal relationships, and normal daily activities.

While there may be a variety of effective methods of treatment for these common ailments, by far the first choice of treatment for most adults is the use of an over-the-counter medicine. These medicines are readily available at every pharmacy, grocery store, and convenience store. They are relatively cheap compared to prescription medicine. But the best thing about OTC medicines is that they usually work well to make people feel better, and in general are quite safe when taken according to the manufacturers' instructions.

Over-the-counter medicines approved by the Food and Drug Administration (FDA) for use must undergo rather rigid safety testing before they can be made available to the general public. This is not true for the so-called "alternative" medicines, supplements, herbal teas, and various other remedies which are on the shelves of most pharmacies and natural food stores.

The major difference between medicines approved by the FDA and alternative products is the scientifically proven efficacy and safety. While some alternative medicines may also be of benefit, there is no control over the purity or quality of these products, their safety and toxicity factors are basically unknown, and their consistent effectiveness is also questionable. (Please see page 25 for further information on herbal medicines in pregnancy.) For this reason, most adults wisely feel safe and comfortable using FDA approved OTC medicines. This concern about safety becomes even more significant when that adult is a pregnant woman.

Chapter Two

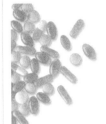

Ingredients In Medications

ACTIVE INGREDIENTS

Non-prescription medications are composed of one or more active ingredients combined with a variety of "inactive ingredients". The active ingredients are always listed on the container. These are always chemical names, frequently unfamiliar, and in this book are referred to as "generic medications". This book only contains information on American OTC medications. Pharmacies from other countries also have a tremendous array of medications which can be purchased without a prescription. However, since regulations on these medications differ from country to country, accurate information on their effectiveness and safety may be hard to get.

Generally, it is the active ingredients which not only work to relieve your symptoms, but are also responsible for concerns about side-effects, allergic reactions, interactions with other medications, and pregnancy-related problems. It is these ingredients which are listed alphabetically in this book for you.

When you purchase an OTC medication during pregnancy, you should always look at the list of active ingredients, even in brand names you use frequently. From time to time, the pharmaceutical companies change the active ingredients but keep the brand name intact, hoping that customers continue to buy their product because of familiarity.

Some containers are so small that the words are readable only with a magnifying glass. If that is the case, the store's pharmacist can help you. Also, you should make sure that there is an expiration date on the label. Past this date, medications begin to lose their effectiveness.

INACTIVE INGREDIENTS

A list of "inactive ingredients" is also written on the containers. The term, "inactive" is sometimes not exactly accurate. In pharmaceutical jargon, "inactive" means that the ingredient does not treat the symptom for which you bought the medicine, but is used primarily for other purposes. These purposes may include: better taste, preservative, lubrication, coloring, etc.

For the most part, these inactive ingredients are benign and helpful. However, significant side-effects and allergic reactions can arise from them as well as from the active ingredients. It is particularly important for women with medical conditions or pregnant women to look at this list as well.

Some of the more concerning inactive ingredients, especially for pregnant women, are sugars, alcohol, Saccharine, aspartame, and caffeine. Others are of minimal significance, unless a person has an allergic reaction to them, which is not uncommon.

Many medicines have a naturally bitter taste and manufacturers may add varying amounts of different kinds of sugar to make them more palatable. They may be listed as dextrose, glucose, fructose, lactose, sucrose, corn syrup, etc. These are all types of sugar.

Pregnant women with diabetes or those who are about to get blood sugar testing may have elevated blood sugar levels when taking these medications.

Saccharine and aspartame are artificial sweeteners and also may be used to improve the flavor of some medicines. Although there has been some concern about saccharine causing bladder cancer in laboratory animals, to date there is no good human evidence that it causes human medical problems when taken appropriately. Aspartame is the chemical found in NutraSweet. It has been exhaustively studied by the FDA. There is no evidence that it causes fetal malformations or newborn problems when taken during pregnancy.

Alcohol is added to some medications to act as a preservative. The amount of alcohol in any one medicine is usually quite small and it is highly doubtful that, when taken according to the manufacturers' suggestions, it could lead to fetal malformations. Nonetheless, if consumed in sufficient quantities, alcohol can lead to a very serious problem for babies, called Fetal Alcohol Syndrome. An additional concern with consuming even very small amounts of alcohol occurs when taking an antibiotic called Metronidazole (common brand name: Flagyl). The combination of these two substances in a person's system may lead to rather severe nausea and vomiting.

The amount of caffeine added as an inactive ingredient in any one medication is usually quite small, perhaps no more than the equivalent of a cup of coffee. This level of caffeine is enough to make a sick person feel a little better, but well short of the amount generally regarded as a concern in pregnancy. Much higher doses of caffeine are related to an increased risk of miscarriage when taken in the first three months of pregnancy.

Other inactive ingredients, such as a variety of lubricants, powders, gels, coloring agents, flavorings, etc. have not been shown to be related to any known pregnancy related problems.

Chapter Three

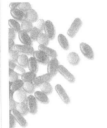

Pregnancy & Medications

P regnant women may have a variety of minor physical ailments which often can be relieved by using OTC medications. Unfortunately, a lack of information along with a fear of potentially causing harm to the developing baby keeps many of them from taking a variety of OTC medicines which may be quite safe. This has resulted in much unnecessary pain and misery for pregnant women.

Pregnant women need to be aware of the potential effects OTC medications may have on them or their developing baby. Some medications are unsafe at any time in pregnancy, some only in early pregnancy, some only in late pregnancy.

This book will provide factual information about the known safety of OTC medications in pregnancy. General information for all adults about effects and side effects of OTC medications can be found in detail in other books (e.g. The Pill Book Guide, The USP Guide to Medicines). The information in this book is generally limited to specific concerns of pregnant women.

Many doctors and nurses are surprised to discover that most OTC medicines appear to be safe in pregnancy. The fear of causing damage to the developing baby, coupled with the fear of being sued should a malformed baby be born, has caused most doctors and nurses to instruct their pregnant patients to avoid all (or nearly all) OTC medicines. This extreme fear of litigation does pregnant women a great disservice. It has led to a national paranoia about medicines in pregnancy which is by and large unnecessary and occasionally seriously harmful.

Using caution is always wise when taking any OTC medication during pregnancy. Before taking them, women may benefit from trying natural methods for relief of symptoms, such as dietary changes for constipation, heat and massage for muscular aches, etc. When these methods are not effective, OTC medicines can often be taken safely if they are taken in the dose recommended and for a brief period of time, usually less than three to five days. If symptoms persist after three days, pregnant women may need to consult their physician.

TIMING IN PREGNANCY

A very important factor in determining any medicine's risk to a developing baby is the gestational age. During the first three months of pregnancy, a baby's organs are in the process of forming. This is the time when developing babies are most susceptible to any damaging effect of outside influences, such as harmful drugs, chemicals, or radiation. After that time has passed, the baby's organs are completely formed and thus the possibility of physical malformations caused by a medication is remote.

When it comes to taking medicine during pregnancy, the most concerning times are the first three months and the last two months. In between those times, roughly from weeks 13 to 32, the risks are minimal, but not completely absent. Theoretically, medications have the potential to affect the functional capabilities of certain organs, most notably the brain, which is developing at a rapid rate throughout pregnancy. The drug well-known for this is alcohol. It is very unlikely that an OTC medication, taken in mid-pregnancy for a few days according to the manufacturers directions, could cause significant problems for a baby. Exceptions are itemized in the discussions of particular medications in the remainder of this book.

The last two months of pregnancy may be of concern primarily because labor may start at any time and a baby whose mother has been taking medications may have a significant amount of that medication in their system after birth. Some types of drugs, especially non-steroidal anti-inflammatory drugs (NSAIDs), which include aspirin and ibuprophen, may have a significant effect on a baby's clotting mechanism or breathing capability and should be avoided during this time. Strong pain medications containing narcotics (which are available only with a prescription) taken in the last few weeks of pregnancy may cause the newborn baby to have serious drug-withdrawal problems. Medications which may increase a mother's blood pressure may worsen a pregnancy-related illness called pre-eclampsia. Before taking any OTC medication in the last few weeks of pregnancy it is generally best to discuss it with your care provider.

Chapter Four

Uncertainties

I n spite of all the scientific studies done to date, there are many unknowns about medications and their potential effects on a baby's future health and development. It is not possible to accurately describe any medication as "perfectly safe" to ANY person, pregnant or not. All medications have at least a very small potential to cause some kind of deleterious side effect.

One of the truly uncertain concerns is a possible future subtle medical effect a medication may have later in childhood or even in adulthood. There are no good scientific data available which show a relationship of any OTC medications to subtle long-term or late onset medical problems.

Even when an individual medication has been shown to be safe in pregnancy, the potential effects on the developing fetus of combinations of medications is completely unknown. As a general rule, it is probably safer to take OTC medications with only one active ingredient than one with many. Some OTC medications are known to affect the absorption of other prescription medicines, reducing their effectiveness. This is especially true of antacids and iron tablets. Women who are taking medicines prescribed by their doctors should consult with them or their pharmacists prior to taking OTC medicines.

Medicine is an ever-changing science. As new research and clinical experience broaden our knowledge, changes in treatment and drug therapy are required. The author has checked with sources believed to be reliable in an effort to provide information that is in accord with the standards accepted at the time of this publication. Readers are advised to check the product information on the package of each drug they plan to use to be certain that the information contained in this work is accurate and that changes have not been made in the ingredients or in contraindications for usage in pregnancy.

Chapter Five

Classification of Drugs in Pregnancy

I n an attempt to clarify the safety of medications in pregnancy, the FDA has assigned risk factors to nearly all drugs based on the level of risk the drug poses to the fetus. When possible, each of the medications listed in this handbook will have a letter next to it (A,B,C,D or X) which corresponds to its risk category. The definitions used for the risk factors are:

CATEGORY A: (Safest)

Controlled studies in women fail to demonstrate a risk to the fetus in the first trimester (and there is no evidence of a risk in later trimesters), and the possibility of fetal harm appears remote.

CATEGORY B:

Either animal-reproduction studies have not demonstrated a fetal risk but there are no controlled studies in pregnant women or animal-reproduction studies have shown an adverse effect (other than a decrease in fertility) that was not confirmed in controlled studies in women in the first trimester (and there is no evidence of a risk in later trimesters).

CATEGORY C:

Either studies in animals have revealed adverse effects on the fetus (teratogenic or embryocidal, or other) and there are no controlled studies in women or studies in women and animals are not available. Drugs should be given only if the potential benefit justifies the potential risk to the fetus.

CATEGORY D:

There is positive evidence of human fetal risk, but the benefits from use in pregnant women may be acceptable despite the risk (e.g., if the drug is needed in a life-threatening situation or for a serious disease for which safer drugs cannot be used or are ineffective).

CATEGORY X:

Studies in animals or human beings have demonstrated fetal abnormalities, or there is evidence of fetal risk based on human experience, or both, and the risk of the use of the drug in pregnant women clearly outweighs any possible benefit. The drug is contraindicated in women who are or may become pregnant.

Occasionally, a drug will have a double designation of risk factors (e.g., Aspirin C/D). The first notation refers to the risk of causing fetal malformations. The second notation refers to other pregnancy related complications which may occur. These are explained in the text with each drug.

Generic medications and the most widely used brand names are listed in this handbook. Many pharmacies have their own brands which are less expensive and usually just as effective as the major brands. It is very important when buying an OTC medication to read the label. Drugs listed as active ingredients on the label are also known as generic medications.

MEDICATIONS TO AVOID

Some OTC medications should probably be avoided throughout pregnancy. The list is surprisingly short. I have included some because of their significant potential for harm and others because their potential for harm is small, but other, safer, equally useful medications are available. These OTC medications are: Aspirin, Bismuth Subsalicylate, Dehydrocholic acid, Ephedrine, Epinephrine, Povidone-Iodine (as a douche), and Phenylephrine (as a decongestant)..

Other medications are a concern only in the first three months of pregnancy and should be avoided at that time. These are: Brompheniramine, Caffeine, and Cimetidine. In the last two months of pregnancy you should avoid: Aspirin (adult strength), Bismuth Subsalicylate, Ibuprofen, Ketoprophen, Naproxyn, and all Salicylates.

Chapter Six

Herbal Medications

Accurate, consistent information about the safety of herbal medications in pregnancy is meager because most have not been studied in a complete scientific manner. In addition, the purity and concentration of any particular herb may vary greatly between manufacturers and even between containers produced by the same manufacturer. The effects of the active chemical compound in one herbal medicine may be altered by diet or other herbal medications resulting in unforseeable results. The same general statement can be applied to many medications called Supplements. Because of these factors, you may see different opinions written on the safety of these substances in pregnancy.

Scientific references have suggested that the following herbs should not be taken during pregnancy:

Aloe
Amaranthus
Angelica
Arnica Grape
Asa Foetida
Asarcum

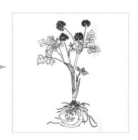

Barberry Root
Barley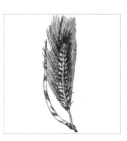
Behen Root
Benzoin Gum Powder
Beth Root
Birthwort
Bittersweet Nightshade
Black Cohosh
Perilla
Black Hellebore
Bladderwrack
Blood Root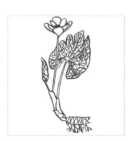
Blue Cohosh
Buchu Leaves (Short Buchu)
Buckthorn Bark
Burdock Root
California Poppy
Camphor
Cascara Sagrada
Castor Oil Plant
Cat's Claw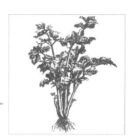
Catnip
Celandine
Celery
Chaste Tree
Chinese Cinnamon
Chinese Motherwort
Chinese Thoroughwax
Chocolate Vine
Cinnamon
Coca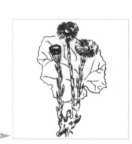
Cocillana Tree
Cola
Colchicum
Colt's Foot

Comfrey
Damiana
Dong Quai
Echinacea
Elder Blossoms
Elecampane
Elephant Ears
English Camomille
English Hawthorn
Ergot

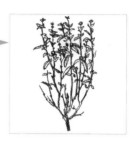

Fennel
Fenugreek
Feverfew
Frangula
German Chamomille
Ginseng
Golden Shower Tree
Goldenseal
Gotu Kola

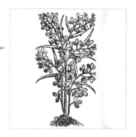

Horehound
Horsemint
Hyssop
Ipecac
Jaborandi
Jack-in-the-Pulpit
Jalap
Jatamansi
Juniper
Kava Kava

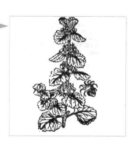

Levant Cotton
Licorice Root
Lilly of the Valley
Lobelia
Lovage
Lycium Bark

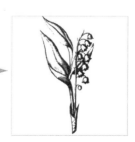

Lycium Berries
Ma Huang (Ephedra)
Maidenhair
Malabar Nut
Male Fern
Mandrake Root
Mayapple
Mexican Scammony Root

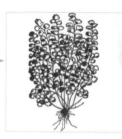

Mistletoe
Mormon Tea
Morning Glory
Motherwort
Mountain Grape
Mugwort
Myrrh
Nutmeg
Orris
Papaya
Parsley Root
Pasque Flower
Pennyroyal Flower

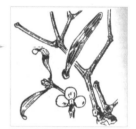

Perilla
Petasites
Pleurisy Root
Poppyseed
Quassia

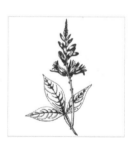

Quinine
Rauwolfia
Rosemary
Rue
Safflower
Saffron
Sage
Saw Palmetto
Scotch Broom

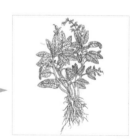

Seneca Snakeroot
Shepherd's Purse
Spikenard
Thuja
Turmeric
Uva-Ursi
Valerian
Vervain
Watercress
White Willow
Wild Indigo
Wormwood
Yew
Zedoary

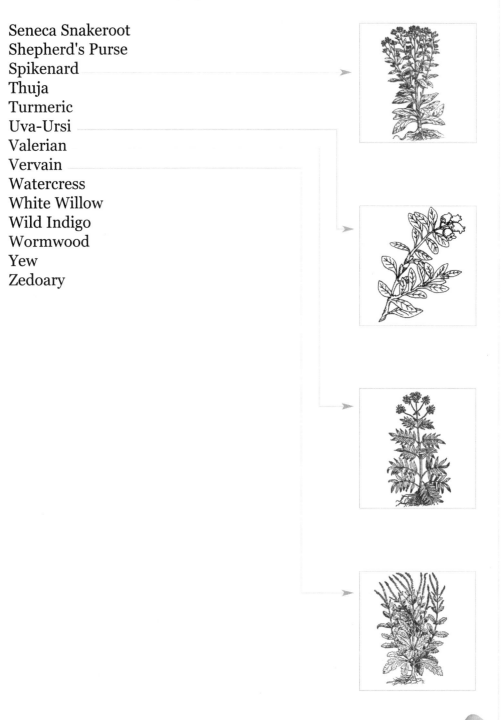

Chapter Seven

Instructions
How to Use this Book

This book is organized such that the generic names of medications are presented alphabetically with their most common brand names, specific pregnancy-related concerns, and comments. If there are additional brand names, an asterisk (*) will signify that these can be found in the appendix beginning on page 145.

There are usually many brand names for each generic medication. In addition, many brands contain more than one generic medication. A good example of this is Robitussin DM, a common cough medication, which contains both Dextromethorphan and Guaifenesin in its formula.

It is generally best to look on the container where it says "active ingredients". There you will find the generic medicines listed. In the index of this book, you then can find that generic name(s) and page(s) where it can be found.

For example, let us say you are interested in knowing about the use and safety of Tylenol in pregnancy. You would look on the box and see that the active ingredient (generic medication) in Tylenol is Acetaminophen. You would then look in the index of this book and be directed to page 35 and find the information under "Acetaminophen".

If you do not have the generic name available, you can also find the page by looking in the index under the brand name. However, not all brands are listed and the formula of some brands may change from year to year making it impossible to keep an accurate up-to-date listing. It is far more reliable to use the generic names listed on the label.

Chapter Eight

Over-the-Counter
Medications in Pregnancy

L isted below are over-the-counter medications and their potential pregnancy related concerns.

* Additional brand names found in appendix

Generic Name:	**ACETAMINOPHEN (B)**
Class of Drug:	Analgesic
Use:	Pain relief
Common Brand Names*:	Tylenol, Liquiprin, Panadol
Pregnancy Related Concerns:	Not known to cause malformations. Considered safe in pregnancy by manufacturers, most physicians, and pharmacists.
Comments:	Acetaminophen is the one analgesic doctors recommend most in pregnancy because of its proven safety record. However, for pregnancy related pain relief, it is usually not as effective as Ibuprofen (see p. 60).

Generic Name:	**ALPHA-GALACTOSIDASE (C)**
Class of Drug:	Anti-Flatulent
Use:	Relief of discomforts of intestinal gas
Common Brand Names:	Beano

Pregnancy Related Concerns: This medicine is an enzyme which, when added to many high fiber foods, breaks their complex sugars into simpler sugars. This transformation makes these foods easier to digest and helps reduce or eliminate gas and bloating. It will make the simple sugars in high fiber foods available to be metabolized by your body. People who are pregnant and who have problems with high blood sugar need to be aware of this potential problem. It may elevate your blood sugar.

Comments: No studies have been done on this medication in early pregnancy, and therefore the potential for causing malformations is unknown, but theoretically very unlikely unless high blood sugars are a concern.

Generic Name:	**ALUMINUM HYDROXIDE**
Class of Drug:	Antacid
Use:	Heartburn relief
Common Brand Names*:	Maalox, Mylanta

Pregnancy Related Concerns: Not known to cause malformations. May decrease absorption of iron.

Most frequent side effect of aluminum antacids is constipation. There is some concern about aluminum and newborn bone growth problems. It is not clear that these antacids are likely to be a problem. However, since there are many effective antacids, it would be wise to avoid frequent use of aluminum hydroxide. Calcium carbonate (see p. 44) is a preferred antacid for most pregnant women because it is more effective and supplies calcium.

ASPIRIN (C/D)

Generic Name:	
Class of Drug:	Analgesic
Use:	Pain relief
Common Brand Names*:	Bayer, St. Joseph, Norwich

Pregnancy Related Concerns: Not known to cause malformations. Use of aspirin in late pregnancy may cause temporary maternal or neonatal bleeding problems. Long-term use is associated with prolonged pregnancy and poor quality contractions in labor.

Comments: No pain relief advantage over acetaminophen. Low dose (baby) aspirin is occasionally beneficial if taken daily for many weeks in certain cases of previous stillborn, under-grown babies, or severe preeclampsia. There is no known harm of baby aspirin; however, your doctor should

37

be the one to decide whether or not you take this. Avoid use of aspirin in pregnancy unless recommended by your physician.

Generic Name:	**ATTAPULGITE (C)**
Class of Drug:	Antidiarrheal
Use:	Relief of diarrhea
Common Brand Names:	Rheaban, Diasorb, Kaopectate, K-Pek

Pregnancy Related Concerns: Very little (if any) of this medicine is absorbed by the body. Therefore, fetal risks or malformations are theoretically very unlikely.

Comments: Premature labor is sometimes associated with diarrhea. Intestinal cramps may, on occasion, be difficult to distinguish from uterine cramps. This medicine will not reduce uterine cramping. If you continue cramping in spite of taking an antidiarrheal medicine, consider the possibility of uterine contractions as the cause of your discomfort and notify your physician or midwife.

Generic Name:	**BACITRACIN (C)**
Class of Drug:	Antibiotic for skin care and first aid
Use:	First aid for cuts, scrapes and bruises
Common Brand Names*:	Baciguent, Neosporin Ointment

Pregnancy Related Concerns: Bacitracin is not known to cause developmental abnormalities in babies. The amount of Bacitracin absorbed through the skin would be extremely small and very unlikely to result in pregnancy related problems.

Generic Name:	**BENZOCAINE (C)**
Class of Drug:	Topical anesthetic
Use:	Relief of minor skin irritaions, Hemorrhoid care
Common Brand Names*:	Lanacane, Solarcaine

Pregnancy Related Concerns: Not known to cause fetal malformations. Very little of this medication is absorbed from the skin so that causing an effect on the developing fetus is very unlikely.

Generic Name:	**BENZOYL PEROXIDE**
Class of Drug:	Skin Care Medication
Use:	Treatment of acne
Common Brand Names*:	Acne-10, Clearasil Maximum Strength Cream, Fostex 10%

Pregnancy Related Concerns: Not known to cause fetal malformations. However, this medication has not been well-studied in pregnancy. The amount of benzoyl peroxide absorbed through the skin and into the maternal circulation is extremely small when it is used after manufacturers recommendations. It is unlikely that the amount of medication absorbed after proper use could have any effect on the developing baby.

Generic Name:	BISACODYL (C)
Class of Drug:	Laxative—Stimulant
Use:	Relief of constipation
Common Brand Names*:	Correctol, Dulcolax, Feen-A-Mint

Pregnancy Related Concerns: Not known to cause fetal malformations. In general, stimulant laxatives are the last resort of treatment for constipation during pregnancy. They should be used rarely. Other methods of constipation relief should be tried first. Dietary changes of increasing fiber and fluid intake, and bulk agent laxatives should be tried prior to using any stimulant laxative. The use of stimulant laxatives will not precipitate labor.

Coments: Avoid stimulant laxatives unless dietary changes and bulk agent laxatives have failed to result in correction of constipation. Chronic use of stimulant laxatives can result in long-standing or permanent bowel dysfunction.

Generic Name:	BISMUTH SUBSALICYLATE (C/D)
Class of Drug:	Antidiarrheal
Use:	Relief of diarrhea
Common Brand Names:	Kaodene NN, Pepto-Bismol, Peptic Relief

Pregnancy Related Concerns: Not known to cause malformations. This medicine is chemically related to aspirin and may cause temporary maternal or newborn bleeding problems, prolonged pregnancy or poor quality contractions in labor. Other, safer medications are available for relief of diarrhea such as loperamide.

Comments: Avoid use of this medicine in pregnancy.

Generic Name: **BROMPHENIRAMINE (C)**
Class of Drug: Antihistamine
Use: Relief of allergy symptoms, additive with many decongestants

Common Brand Names*: Bromfed, Dimetapp, Drixoral Cold and Flu.

Pregnancy Related Concerns: There is a weak association with some congenital defects with the use of brompheniramine. Also, rarely, very premature babies whose mothers have taken antihistamines just prior to premature delivery have had an eye disorder (retrolental fibroplasia). This precaution is for all antihistamines.

Comments: Avoid use of this medicine in the first three months of pregnancy. Avoid daily use in the last three months of pregnancy if premature labor is a concern.

Generic Name: **BUTOCONAZOLE (C)**
Class of Drug: Vaginal antifungal agent
Use: Relief of vaginal yeast infections

41

Common Brand Names:	Femstat-3, Mycelex-3

Pregnancy Related Concerns: Not known to cause malformations. There are no known specific fetal concerns. However, symptoms of a yeast infection of the vagina may be confused with other infectious problems. Also, diabetes may lead to frequent yeast infections.

Comments: This medication is commonly used for treatment of vaginal yeast infections during pregnancy. However, if symptoms persist, or the problem is recurrent, you should discuss this with your doctor.

Generic Name:	**CAFFEINE (B)**
Class of Drug:	Stimulant
Use:	Stimulant
Common Brand Names*:	20/20, Caffedrine, Vivarin

Pregnancy Related Concerns: The frequent use of high doses of caffeine in early pregnancy is related to an increased risk of miscarriages. The amount of caffeine in these pills is considerably more than that found in coffee, tea, or cola drinks. This medicine is found in much smaller amounts as an additive in a variety of other medicines and in those smaller doses is considered harmless for a developing baby.

Comments: Caffeine taken as a medication should be used rarely if ever during pregnancy. Consumed by breastfeeding mothers, caffeine may lead to irritable babies who sleep poorly. The amount of caffeine in two or three cans of caffeinated soft drinks or cups of coffee per day has not been associated with significant fetal problems.

Generic Name:	**CALAMINE**
Class of Drug:	Topical Anti-Irritant
Use:	Relief from itching
Common Brand Names*:	Aveeno Anti-Itch, Caladryl

Pregnancy Related Concerns: When used on the skin, calamine is not absorbed from the skin and therefore has little potential for affecting the baby in any way.

Comments: Calamine may be helpful late in pregnancy if skin itching becomes an annoyance.

Generic Name:	**CALCIUM**
Class of Drug:	Dietary Supplement
Use:	Mineral
Common Brand Names*:	Caltrate, Os-Cal 500, Tums

Pregnancy Related Concerns: Calcium is needed during pregnancy for the formation of fetal bones. In order to provide that calcium, there is a natural increase in the absorption of calcium from the intestines during pregnancy. The amount of calcium the baby requires is easily provided by the mother, even when dietary

43

calcium intake is sub-optimal. Although calcium supplementation is often suggested by a variety of well-meaning health care providers, there is no evidence that it is necessary during pregnancy for most healthy American women. Too much oral calcium can lead to nausea, vomiting, weakness, headaches, poor diet, constipation, and an increase in intestinal gas.

Comments: Avoid the unnecessary use of supplemental calcium unless you have a very specific medical condition which requires its use.

CALCIUM CARBONATE AND CALCIUM CARBIMIDE

Generic Name:
Class of Drug: Antacid
Use: Heartburn relief
Common Brand Names*: Alka-Mints, Rolaids Calcium Rich, Titralac, Tums

Pregnancy Related Concerns: Not known to cause malformations. Too much calcium can lead to nausea, vomiting, weakness, headaches, poor diet, constipation, and an increase in intestinal gas. Women with significant kidney disorders are more likely to have these problems.

Comments: This medication is the one preferred by most pregnant women with heartburn. It is not only effective, but it

44

lasts longer and provides a good source of additional calcium.

Generic Name:	**CALCIUM POLYCARBOPHIL**
Class of Drug:	Laxative—Bulk Agent
Use:	Relief of constipation
Common Brand Names:	FiberCon, Konsyl Fiber, FiberNorm, Equalactin

Pregnancy Related Concerns: Very little if any of this medication is absorbed from the intestinal system. Therefore, the possibility that it could affect a baby is remote.

Comments: Constipation is a very frequent problem in pregnancy. The first step in treating constipation in pregnancy is to increase dietary fiber and fluids. Only if that is unsuccessful should laxative products be considered. Bulking agents are the next logical step for relief of constipation if dietary changes prove unsuccessful. It is important to use this and all laxatives very sporadically and only as needed. Some medications containing bulk agents have a great deal of sugar in them which may affect the blood sugar levels of women who have diabetes during pregnancy.

Generic Name:	**CAMPHOR (C)**
Class of Drug:	Topical analgesic, cough suppressant
Use:	Relief of muscular and joint pain, relief of minor cough.

Common Brand Names*:   Heet, Noxzema Medicated Skin Cream, Vicks Cough Drops, Vicks VapoRub

Pregnancy Related Concerns: Not known to cause malformations or pregnancy-related problems. Very little information is available on its safety in pregnancy.

Generic Name: **CAPSAICIN (C)**
Class of Drug: Topical Analgesic
Use: Relief of muscular and joint pain
Common Brand Names*:   Capzasin-P, Pain Doctor, Rid-a-Pain, Sloan's, Zostrix

Pregnancy Related Concerns: Not known to cause malformations or other pregnancy related problems. Very little information is available on its safety in pregnancy.

Generic Name: **CASANTHRANOL (C)**
Class of Drug: Laxative-Stimulant
Use: Relief of constipation
Common Brand Names*:   Genasoft Plus, Peri-Colace, Peri-Dos, Pro-Sof

Pregnancy Related Concerns: Not known to cause fetal malformations. In general, stimulant laxatives are the last resort of treatment for constipation during pregnancy. These should be used rarely. Other methods of constipation relief should be tried first. Dietary changes of increasing fiber and fluid intake, and bulk agent laxatives should be tried prior to using any stimulant laxative.

The use of stimulant laxatives will not precipitate labor.

Comments: Avoid stimulant laxatives unless dietary changes and bulk agent laxatives have failed to result in correction of constipation. Chronic use of stimulant laxatives can result in long-standing or permanent bowel dysfunction.

Generic Name: **CASCARA (C)**
Class of Drug: Laxative—Stimulant
Use: Relief of constipation
Common Brand Names*: Bilstan, Cascara Aromatic, Nature's Remedy.

Pregnancy Related Concerns: Not known to cause fetal malformations. In general, stimulant laxatives are the last resort of treatment for constipation during pregnancy. These should be used rarely. Other methods of constipation relief should be tried first. Dietary changes of increasing fiber and fluid intake, and bulk agent laxatives should be tried prior to using any stimulant laxative. The use of stimulant laxatives will not precipitate labor.

Comments: Avoid stimulant laxatives unless dietary changes and bulk agent laxatives have failed to result in correction of constipation. Chronic use of stimulant laxatives can result in long-standing or permanent bowel dysfunction.

Generic Name: **CASTOR OIL**
Class of Drug: Laxative—Stimulant
Use: Relief of constipation
Common Brand Names: Emulsoil, Neoloid, Purge

Pregnancy Related Concerns: Not known to cause fetal malformations. In general, stimulant laxatives are the last resort of treatment for constipation during pregnancy. These should be used rarely. Dietary changes of increasing fiber and fluid intake, and bulk agent laxatives should be tried prior to using any stimulant laxative. The use of stimulant laxatives will not precipitate labor.

Comments: Avoid stimulant laxatives unless dietary changes and bulk agent laxatives have failed to result in correction of constipation. Chronic use of stimulant laxatives can result in long-standing or permanent bowel dysfunction.

Generic Name: **CHARCOAL**
Class of Drug: Antidote, Antiflatulent
Use: Relieve discomforts of intestinal gas
Common Brand Names: CharcoAid, Charcoal Plus, Charco Caps, LiquiChar

Pregnancy Related Concerns: Not known to cause fetal malformations.

Comments: This is a relatively inert medication which does not enter the blood stream and therefore very unlikely to affect a growing baby.

Generic Name: CHLORPHENIRAMINE (B)
Class of Drug: Antihistamine
Use: Relief of allergy symptoms, additive with many decongestants
Common Brand Names*: Chlor-Trimeton Allergy Tablets, Sinarest Extra Strength, Triaminic Cold & Allergy

Pregnancy Related Concerns: Not known to cause malformations. In fact, scientific data actually show a lower risk to babies whose mothers took this medicine compared to controls. Rarely, very premature babies whose mothers have taken antihistamines just prior to delivery have had eye disorders (retrolental fibroplasia). This precaution is for all antihistamines.

Comments: Found in a wide variety of combination medications for relief of cold symptoms. Avoid daily use in the last three months of pregnancy if premature labor is a concern.

Generic Name: CIMETIDINE (B)
Class of Drug: Histamine H2-receptor antagonist, antacid
Use: Relief of heartburn
Common Brand Names: Tagamet HB

49

Pregnancy Related Concerns: Not known to cause fetal malformations. This medication has a very mild anti-androgenic effect. This means that there is a theoretical concern that it could affect the masculinization of a male fetus if taken early in pregnancy. Other medicines of this class do not have this problem. This medication may change the effectiveness of a variety of prescription medications. This concern should be discussed with a physician or pharmacist. When taking certain antacids, the effectiveness of cimetidine is decreased.

Comments: If antacids alone are insufficient for relief of heartburn symptoms, this type of medication often works very well. There are other medications of this class that work just as well without the anti-androgen concern. Therefore, use famotidine, nizatidine or ranitidine instead of cimetidine. Most pediatricians recommend avoiding use of cimetidine while breastfeeding as it may affect the baby's stomach acid production.

Generic Name: **CLEMASTINE (C)**
Class of Drug: Antihistamine
Use: Relief of allergy symptoms
Common Brand Names: Tavist Allergy, Dayhist-1

Pregnancy Related Concerns: Not known to cause malformations.

Rarely, very premature babies whose mothers have taken antihistamines just prior to delivery have had eye disorders (retrolental fibroplasia). This precaution is for all antihistamines.

Comments:

The American Academy of Pediatrics cautions that use in mothers who are breastfeeding may result in drowsy or irritable babies (based on a single case report). Avoid daily use in the last three months of pregnancy if premature labor is a concern.

CLOTRIMAZOLE (B)

Generic Name:
Class of Drug: Antifungal agent for vaginal or skin infections

Use: Treatment of vaginal and skin yeast infections

Common Brand Names: Desenex Cream, Gyne-Lotrimin, Lotrimin, Lotrimin AF, Mycelex

Pregnancy Related Concerns: Not known to cause malformations. Symptoms of a yeast infection of the vagina may be confused with other infectious problems. Also, diabetes may lead to frequent yeast infections.

Comments: See your doctor before using this medicine repeatedly for vaginal infections to make sure you are treating the problem correctly.

Generic Name:	COAL TAR
Class of Drug:	Keratolytic agent
Use:	Treatment of dandruff, seborrhea and psoriasis
Common Brand Names*:	Denorex, Psorigel

Pregnancy Related Concerns: When used according to manufacturers' directions, no pregnancy related problems have been reported. There is little, if any, of this medication absorbed from the skin.

Generic Name:	DEHYDROCHOLIC ACID
Class of Drug:	Laxative—Stimulant
Use:	Relief of constipation
Common Brand Names:	Atrocholin, Cholan-DH, Decholin

Pregnancy Related Concerns: Dehydrocholic acid is one of the few laxative stimulants which is absorbed by the body and has the potential to cross the placenta and get into fetal circulation. It is not known whether this medication will affect the baby significantly.

Comments: If a stimulant laxative is to be used, avoid this one.

Generic Name:	DEXTROMETHORPHAN(DM) (C)
Class of Drug:	Cough Medicine
Use:	Relief from cough symptoms
Common Brand Names*:	Robitussin DM, Vicks 44 Cough Relief

Pregnancy Related Concerns: Not known to cause human malformations or other pregnancy related problems. Because it is usually combined with other medicines, it is difficult to isolate concerns about DM scientifically. There may be alcohol in some of these cough syrups. While fetal alcohol syndrome is a concern during pregnancy, the amount of alcohol consumed by using cough medicine for a few days is too small to significantly affect the growing baby.

Comments: Occasional use of cough medicine with DM in pregnancy has not been reported to cause newborn problems. Do not exceed recommended dose. DM works by inhibiting the cough mechanism. If you need to take DM for more than five consecutive days, you may be having a significant medical problem and should contact your doctor.

Generic Name: DIBUCAINE
Class of Drug: Local anesthetic
Use: Relief of minor skin irritations, Hemorrhoid care
Common Brand Names: Nupercainal, Nupercaine, Otocort

Pregnancy Related Concerns: Not known to cause fetal malformations or other pregnancy related problems when used according to the manufacturers' directions.

Generic Name: DIMENHYDRINATE (B)
Class of Drug: Antihistamine

53

Use: Relief of allergy symptoms, relief of
                                  nausea, sleep aid
Common Brand Names: Dramamine, Traveltabs

Pregnancy Related Concerns: Not known to cause malformations.
                                  Rarely, very premature babies whose
                                  mothers have taken antihistamines
                                  just prior to delivery have had eye
                                  disorders (retrolental fibroplasia).

Comments: This medicine makes a person
                                  sleepy. Avoid daily use in the last
                                  three months of pregnancy if prema-
                                  ture labor is a concern. This medi-
                                  cine works well for nausea due to
                                  motion sickness.

Generic Name: ## DIPHENHYDRAMINE (C)
Class of Drug: Antihistamine
Use: Relief of allergy symptoms, relief of
                                  nausea, sleep aid, additive with many
                                  decongestants, relief of skin itching
                                  late in pregnancy
Common Brand Names*:   Benadryl, Sominex, Unisom with
                                  Pain Relief

Pregnancy Related Concerns: Not known to cause malformations.
                                  Rarely, very premature babies whose
                                  mothers have taken antihistamines
                                  just prior to delivery have had eye
                                  disorders (retrolental fibroplasia).
                                  This precaution is for all antihista-
                                  mines. Very high doses of diphen-
                                  hydramine may lead to uterine

contractions or withdrawal symptoms in a newborn.

Comments: Diphenhydramine may be used early in pregnancy for relief of nausea. Avoid daily use in the last three months of pregnancy if premature delivery is a concern. This medicine makes a person sleepy. When getting to sleep is difficult late in pregnancy, 25 mg of diphenhydramine at bedtime can be very helpful when all else fails. It is commonly suggested as a treatment for itching in late pregnancy.

Generic Name: DOCUSATE SALTS (Docusate calcium, Docusate sodium) (C)

Class of Drug: Laxative—Stool Softener

Use: Relief of constipation

Common Brand Names*: Colace, Correctol Extra Gentle

Pregnancy Related Concerns: Not known to cause fetal malformations. Very little of this medicine is absorbed from the intestinal system and therefore potential effects on the growing baby are considered only remotely possible.

Comments: As with all laxative bulk agents and softeners, this medicine should be taken only sporadically. Increasing dietary fiber and fluids should be the first step in controlling constipation problems.

Generic Name: **DOXYLAMINE (A)**

Class of Drug: Antihistamine

Use: Relief of nausea and vomiting of pregnancy, allergy symptoms, additive with many decongestants, sleep aid

Common Brand Names*: Unisom Night-Time Sleep Aid, Vicks NyQuil Cough Liquid

Pregnancy Related Concerns: Not known to cause malformations. Rarely, very premature babies whose mothers have taken antihistamines just prior to premature delivery have develeped an eye disorder (retrolental fibroplasia).

Comments: Combined with vitamin B6, taken at bedtime, this medicine works very nicely to reduce the nausea and vomiting of early pregnancy. This medicine makes a person sleepy. Avoid daily use in the last three months of pregnancy if premature labor is a concern.

Generic Name: **EPHEDRINE (C)**

Class of Drug: Decongestant, Bronchodilator

Use: Relief of nasal and sinus congestion due to colds

Common Brand Names: Bronkaid Dual Action, Dynafed Asthma Relief, Primatene

Pregnancy Related Concerns: Products containing ephedrine may increase a woman's blood pressure as well as decreasing blood flow to the uterus and developing baby. Safety in the first 13 weeks is questionable.

Comments: Avoid frequent use of this medication throughout pregnancy.

Generic Name: **EPINEPHRINE (C)**
Class of Drug: Bronchodilator
Use: Treatment of asthma
Common Brand Names: MicroNefrin, Primatene Mist

Pregnancy Related Concerns: Epinephrine has been shown to increase blood pressure and decrease blood flow to the uterus. There is evidence that it may cause inguinal hernias in babies.

Comments: Avoid frequent use of this medicine in pregnancy. There are many other excellent, safe medicines for asthma. If you need one, ask your doctor for a prescription for one of them.

Generic Name: **FAMOTIDINE (B)**
Class of Drug: Histamine H2-receptor antagonist, antacid
Use: Relief of heartburn
Common Brand Names: Pepcid

Pregnancy Related Concerns: Not known to cause malformations. This medication may change the effectiveness of a variety of prescription medications. This concern should be discussed with a physician or pharmacist. When taking certain antacids, the effectiveness of famotidine is decreased.

Comments:

If antacids alone are insufficient for relief of heartburn symptoms, this type of medication often works very well. It works best if taken twice a day. Do not take antacids at the same time. Most pediatricians recommend avoiding use of famotidine while breastfeeding as it may affect the baby's stomach acid production.

Generic Name:
Class of Drug:
Use:
Pregnancy Related Concerns:

FOLIC ACID (A)
Dietary Supplement
Nutritional supplement
Folic acid is a vitamin which has a major influence in two separate areas of interest in pregnancy: prevention of some fetal defects and formation of blood cells. There is growing evidence that supplementation of the maternal diet with folic acid prior to pregnancy and during the first three months of pregnancy may reduce the risk of spinal defects and possibly other abnormalities as well. Folic acid taken after the third month of pregnancy would not be expected to have any beneficial effect on fetal formation. Later in pregnancy, some women develop anemia due to a low folic acid intake. This anemia can almost always be quickly and easily cured by taking folic acid tablets.

Comments:

For most women anticipating a pregnancy—take 0.4 mg of folic acid daily for at least a month prior to pregnancy and for the first three months of the pregnancy. For those women who have previously had a baby with a neural tube defect—increase that dose to 4 mg of folic acid a day.

Generic Name:	**GUAIFENESIN (C)**
Class of Drug:	Cough Medicines
Use:	Expectorant, Loosens respiratory tract secretions
Common Brand Names*:	Anti-Tuss, Robitussin, Wal-Tussin DM

Pregnancy Related Concerns: Not known to cause malformations or other pregnancy related problems. This medicine is found in many over-the-counter cough medicines alone or in combination with dextromethorphan.

Comments: If you need to take this medicine for more than five days, you may be having a significant medical problem and should contact your doctor.

Generic Name:	**HYDROCORTISONE(TOPICAL)**
Class of Drug:	Skin care medication, topical steroid
Use:	Relief of skin irritations
Common Brand Names*:	Anusol HC, Cortaid, Lanacort, Hydrocortisone 1%

Pregnancy Related Concerns: The amount of hydrocortisone in skin care preparations which is absorbed into the circulation is extremely small. It is doubtful that the fetus could be exposed to any sig-nificant amount of hydrocortisone from proper use of these topical medications. As always, it is appro-priate to follow the directions given by the manufacturer.

Comments: It is important that this medication not be used for sore skin around nip-ples during breastfeeding, because the baby may absorb this.

Generic Name: **IBUPROFEN (B/D)**
Class of Drug: Analgesic
Use: Pain relief
Common Brand Names*: Advil, Midol Maximum Strength, Motrin IB

Pregnancy Related Concerns: Not known to cause malformations. This medication has the theoretical potential to cause temporary mater-nal or neonatal coagulation prob-lems, but these are rare. May cause serious problems after 32 weeks with fetal circulation and urine produc-tion. May prolong pregnancy if taken daily.

Comments: Ibuprofen is occasionally recom-mended to reduce contractions before 32 weeks. It is an excellent medication for relief of minor pains in pregnancy when used sporadically prior to 32 weeks. It is more effective than acetaminophen for the types of pain pregnant women experience.

Heartburn may be an aggravating side effect. If you need to use this medicine more than three times a day for more than three to five days, you should contact your physician. Avoid use of ibuprofen in the last eight weeks of pregnancy.

Generic Name:	**IRON (FERROUS FUMARATE, FERROUS GLUCONATE, FERROUS SULFATE)**
Class of Drug:	Nutritional supplement, mineral
Use:	Production of red blood cells and hemoglobin
Common Brand Names*:	Ferro-Sequels, Feosol, Fero-Folic 500, Slo Fe

Pregnancy Related Concerns: Requirements for iron increase significantly during pregnancy, especially in the last four months. Supplementation with medicinal iron may be necessary for many, but not all pregnant women. Because iron requirements are less during the first half of pregnancy, additional iron may not be needed during that time. Iron tablets frequently result in annoying side effects of nausea, vomiting, and/or constipation, especially early in pregnancy when women are more susceptible to these problems anyway. Most prenatal vitamins contain iron. Taking these may result in worsening of gastrointestinal side effects.

Comments:	Unless you are known to have an iron-deficiency problem, avoid use of iron supplementation of the first half of the pregnancy. Most pregnant women will receive sufficient supplemental iron with one iron tablet per day thereafter. Iron-containing medicine has been a frequent source of poisoning for small children who have ingested large numbers of these tablets. Keep this medicine away from the reach of small children.

Generic Name:	**KAOLIN (C)**
Class of Drug:	Antidiarrheal
Use:	Relief of diarrhea
Common Brand Names*:	Kaopectate, Kapectin

Pregnancy Related Concerns:	Very little (if any) of this medicine is absorbed by the body. Therefore, risks of malformations are theoretically very unlikely.

Comments:	Premature labor is sometimes associated with diarrhea. Intestinal cramps may, on occasion, be difficult to distinguish from uterine cramps. This medicine will not reduce uterine cramping. If you continue cramping in spite of taking an antidiarrheal medicine, consider the possibility of uterine contractions as the cause of your discomfort and notify your physician or midwife.

Generic Name: **KETOPROFEN**
Class of Drug: Analgesic
Use: Pain relief
Common Brand Names: Orudis KT

Pregnancy Related Concerns: Not known to cause malformations. This medication has the theoretical potential to cause temporary maternal or neonatal coagulation problems, but these are rare. May cause serious problems after 32 weeks with fetal circulation and urine production. May prolong pregnancy if taken daily.

Comments: Ketoprofen may be used sporadically for pain relief before 32 weeks. Heartburn may be an aggravating side effect. If you need to use this medicine more than three times a day for more than three to five days, you should contact your physician. Avoid use of ketoprofen in the last eight weeks of pregnancy.

Generic Name: **LACTASE**
Class of Drug: Digestive Enzyme
Use: Aids in digestion of dairy foods
Common Brand Names: Dairy Ease, LactAid, Lactrase, SureLac

Pregnancy Related Concerns: Not known to cause fetal malformations. However, this medication breaks down complex sugars in the intestines and may increase blood sugar levels. This is of particular importance for women with diabetes or those about to get blood sugar tests.

Comments: This medicine may be very helpful for women who have difficulty digesting dairy products. Many dairy products provide important nutrients in pregnancy. This medication will allow pregnant women with lactose intolerance to get those nutritional benefits. Be sure to inform your midwife or doctor that you are taking this medication as it may increase your blood sugars.

Generic Name: **LIDOCAINE (TOPICAL)**
Class of Drug: Topical anesthetic
Use: Relief of minor skin irritations
Common Brand Names: Dermaflex, ELA-Max, Solarcaine Aloe Extra Burn Relief, TheraPatch Cold Sore, Zilactin-L

Pregnancy Related Concerns: Not known to cause fetal malformations or other pregnancy related problems when used according to the manufacturers' directions.

Generic Name: **LINDANE (B)**
Class of Drug: Pediculocide
Use: Treatment of lice infestation
Common Brand Names: Kwell, Lindane Lotion and Shampoo

Pregnancy Related Concerns: Small amounts of this medication are absorbed through intact skin and mucous membranes. It has the small potential to produce toxic effects on nerves. There has been no direct evidence that the use of lindane during pregnancy has resulted in fetal malformations.

Comments:

The manufacturer recommends using lindane no more than twice during a pregnancy. Because of lindane's potentially serious toxicity, treatment of lice infestations during pregnancy is best done with pyrethrins with piperonyl butoxide (see p. 81).

Generic Name: **LOPERAMIDE (B)**

Class of Drug: Antidiarrheal

Use: Relief of diarrhea

Common Brand Names*: Imodium A-D, K-Pek II, Neo-Diaral

Pregnancy Related Concerns: Not known to cause malformations. Premature labor is sometimes associated with diarrhea. Intestinal cramps may, on occasion, be difficult to distinguish from uterine cramping. If you continue cramping in spite of taking this medicine, consider the possibility of uterine contractions as the cause of your discomfort and notify your midwife or doctor.

Comments:

This is an effective medication for most cases of mild diarrhea. Do not take more than the dosage listed on the label. Do not take more than one dose if you are in early labor, as there is a small chance of causing neonatal respiratory depression if the baby is born shortly after using this type of medication.

Generic Name:	**LORATADINE**
Class of Drug:	Antihistamine
Use:	Relief of allergy symptoms
Common Brand Names:	Claritin

Pregnancy Related Concerns: Not known to cause fetal malformations. However, long-term information on babies whose mothers have taken this medicine is not available.

Comments: This medication has not had the extensive evaluation and scientific study in pregnancy which other antihistamines have undergone. Other antihistamines (e.g., chlorpheniramine) may be a safer choice in the first three months of pregnancy. Loratidine works well with fewer side-effects than most OTC antihistamines and may be a good choice beyond the first trimester. At this time it is also much more expensive than other OTC antihistamines.

Generic Name:	**MAGALDRATE**
Class of Drug:	Antacid
Use:	Heartburn Relief
Common Brand Names:	Losopan, Lowsium, Riopan

Pregnancy Related Concerns: Not known to cause fetal malforma- tions. May decrease absorption of iron. Most frequent side effect is con- stipation. There are other, more effective antacids with fewer side effects. Calcium carbonate (see p. 42) is favored by many pregnant women because it is very effective, lasts longer, and supplies additional calcium.

Generic Medication: **MAGNESIUM SALICYLATE—** See Salicylates p. 84.

Generic Name: **MAGNESIUM SALTS** (magnesium aluminate, magnesium carbonate, magnesium gluconate, magnesium hydroxide, magnesium trisilicate) (B)

Class of Drug: Antacid, Laxative

Use: Heartburn relief, constipation relief

Common Brand Names*: Di-Gel, Gaviscon, Maalox, Mylanta, Phillips' Milk of Magnesia

Pregnancy Related Concerns: Not known to cause malformations. Repeated doses can cause diarrhea and fluid imbalances. Women with severe kidney disorders may suffer serious consequences from taking this medication.

Comments: This medicine may be used sporadi- cally, but is not advised for long-term use in pregnancy. A more effective antacid during pregnancy is calcium carbonate (see p. 44) which also provides an additional source of calcium.

Generic Name: **MALT**
Class of Drug: Laxative—Bulk agent
Use: Relief of constipation
Common Brand Names: Maltsupex, Syllamalt

Pregnancy Related Concerns: Very little if any of bulk agents is absorbed from the intestinal system. Therefore, the possibility that they could affect a baby is remote.

Comments: Constipation is a very frequent problem in pregnancy. The first step in treating constipation in pregnancy is to increase dietary fiber and fluids. Only if that is unsuccessful should laxative products be considered. Bulking agents are the next logical step for relief of constipation if dietary changes prove unsuccessful. It is important to use this and all laxatives very sporadically and only as needed. Some medications containing bulk agents have a great deal of sugar in them which may increase the blood sugar levels of women who have diabetes during pregnancy.

Generic Name: **MECLIZINE (B)**
Class of Drug: Antihistamine
Use: Nausea relief, sleep aid
Common Brand Names: Bonine, Dramamine II

Pregnancy Related Concerns: Not known to cause malformations. Rarely, very premature babies whose mothers have taken antihistamines just prior to delivery have had eye disorders (retrolental fibroplasia). This medicine makes a person sleepy.

Comments:

This medicine may be very effective for relief of nausea in early pregnancy. Avoid daily use in the last three months of pregnancy if premature labor is a concern.

Generic Name: **MENTHOL**
Class of Drug: Cough medicine, local anesthesia
Use: Relief of cough and sore throat symptoms
Common Brand Names*:   Cepacol Anesthetic Lozenges, Isodettes, N'Ice 'N Clear, Sucrets 4-Hour Cough, Vicks Cough Drops

Pregnancy Related Concerns: Not known to cause malformations or other pregnancy related problems. Very little information is available on the safety of this medication in pregnancy.

Comments:

Menthol is frequently combined with eucalyptus oil for temporary relief of sore throats and cough. Do not exceed manufacturers' recommendations.

Generic Name: **METHYLCELLULOSE**
Class of Drug: Laxative—Bulk Agent
Use: Relief of constipation
Common Brand Names: Citrucel, Citrucel Sugar Free

Pregnancy Related Concerns: Very little if any of bulk agents is absorbed from the intestinal system. Therefore, the possibility that they could affect a baby is remote.

Comments: Constipation is a very frequent problem in pregnancy. The first step in treating constipation in pregnancy is to increase dietary fiber and fluids. Only if that is unsuccessful should laxative products be considered. Bulking agents are the next logical step for relief of constipation if dietary changes prove unsuccessful. It is important to use this and all laxatives very sporadically and only as needed. Some medications containing bulk agents have a great deal of sugar in them which may increase the blood sugar levels of women who have diabetes during pregnancy.

Generic Medication: METHYL SALICYLATE (See Salicylates p. 84)

Generic Name: MICONAZOLE (C)
Class of Drug: Antifungal agent for vaginal or skin infections
Use: Treatment of vaginal and skin yeast infections
Common Brand Names: Micatin, Monistat

Pregnancy Related Concerns: Not known to cause malformations. There are no known specific fetal concerns. However, symptoms of a yeast infection of the vagina may be confused with other infectious problems. Also, diabetes may lead to frequent yeast infections.

Comments:

This medication is commonly used for vaginal yeast infections during pregnancy. However, if symptoms persist, or if the problem is recurrent, you should discuss this with your doctor.

Generic Name: **MINERAL OIL**
Class of Drug: Laxative—stool softener
Use: Relief of constipation
Common Brand Names: Fleet Mineral Oil, Kondremul Plain, Liqui-Doss, Milkinol, Petrolatum

Pregnancy Related Concerns: Very little of this medicine is absorbed from the intestinal system and therefore potential effects on the growing baby are considered only remotely possible.

Comments:

As with all laxative bulk agents and softeners, this medicine should be taken only sporadically. Increasing dietary fiber and fluids should be the first step in controlling constipation problems.

Generic Name: **NAPHAZOLINE HYDROCHLORIDE**
Class of Drug: Decongestant
Use: Relief of nasal congestion; relief of itching and irritation of the eyes due to allergies

Common Brand Names*: Allerest Eye Drops, Clear Eyes, Naphcon A

Pregnancy Related Concerns: No known pregnancy related problems when taken according to manufacturers' suggestions.

Comments: Do not use this medicine for more than three consecutive days because a rebound worsening of congestion may occur.

Generic Name: **NAPROXYN (B/D)**
Class of Drug: Non-steroidal anti-inflammatory drug, analgesic
Use: Pain relief
Common Brand Names: Aleve, Naprosyn

Pregnancy Related Concerns: Not known to cause malformations. Has the theoretical potential to cause temporary maternal or neonatal coagulation problems, but these are rare. May cause serious problems after 32 weeks with fetal circulation and urine production. May prolong pregnancy if taken daily.
Naproxyn may be used sporadically for pain relief before 32 weeks.

Comments: Heartburn may be an aggravating side effect. If you need to use this medicine more than three times a day for more than three to five days, you should contact your physician. Avoid use of naproxyn in the last eight weeks of pregnancy.

Generic Name:	**NEOMYCIN (C)**
Class of Drug:	Antibiotic
Use:	First aid for cuts, scrapes, burns and skin infections
Common Brand Names*:	Lanabiotic, Neosporin

Pregnancy Related Concerns: Neomycin is an antibiotic which is chemically related to the antibiotics gentamicin, kanamycin, strepto-mycin, and tobramycin. These other antibiotics have been associated with damage to the eighth cranial nerve in fetuses resulting in hearing loss. Although neomycin itself has never been directly implicated in cases of hearing loss when used during pregnancy, theoretically that potential does exist. The amount of neomycin absorbed through the skin will vary with medication, length of use, and frequency of use. Nonetheless, enough neomycin could potentially be absorbed through the skin to cause fetal problems if used frequently. Occasional use is not likely to cause newborn problems.

Comments: Avoid frequent use of neomycin antibiotic creams during pregnancy for first aid and skin infections unless instructed by your physician. Use other topical antibiotics such as bacitracin or polymyxin if frequent use is needed.

Generic Name:
Class of Drug:
Use:
Common Brand Names:

NICOTINE (D)
Smoking Cessation Products
Assist in smoking cessation
Habitrol, Nicoderm, Nicorette Gum, Nicotrol, Prostep

Pregnancy Related Concerns: Smoking during pregnancy results in a higher risk for a variety of poor pregnancy outcomes. There is no doubt that smoking is a bad thing to do during pregnancy. Unfortunately, these products all contain nicotine which is one of the major chemicals absorbed by the body during smoking. Nicotine all by itself is potentially harmful to the developing baby and it has been shown that the use of these medications results in a rather high nicotine level in the bloodstream during pregnancy.

Comments: Use of these products provides less nicotine than cigarette smoking. If the choice is smoking or nicotine use, the latter is generally safer.

Generic Name:
Class of Drug:

Use:
Common Brand Names:

NIZATIDINE (C)
Histamine H2 receptor antagonist, antacid
Relief of heartburn
Axid

Pregnancy Related Concerns: Not known to cause malformations. This medication may change the effectiveness of a variety of prescription medications. This concern should be discussed with a physician or pharmacist. When taking certain antacids, the effectiveness of nizatidine is decreased.

Comments:

If antacids alone are insufficient for relief of heartburn symptoms, these types of medications often work very well. It works best if taken twice a day. Do not take antacids at the same time. Most pediatricians recommend avoiding use of nizatidine while breastfeeding as it may affect the baby's gastric acid secretion.

Generic Name: NONOXYNOL-9

Class of Drug: Spermicide

Use: Prevention of pregnancy

Common Brand Names: Advantage 24, Conceptrol, Delfen, Emko, Encare, Gynol II, K-Y Plus, Koromex, Ortho-Gynol, Semicid Inserts, Shur-Seal, VCF

Pregnancy Related Concerns: This medicine has been extensively studied and is not felt to be related to fetal malformations or other pregnancy related problems.

Comments: Initial information indicated that nonoxynol-9 may reduce the transmission of the HIV virus. That has not proven to be true and therefore, there is no reason to use this medicine after the pregnancy has begun.

Generic Name: OXYMETAZOLINE HYDROCHLORIDE
Class of Drug: Decongestant
Use: Relief of nasal congestion, relief of eye irritation due to allergies
Common Brand Names*:   Afrin Nasal Spray, Dristan 12-Hour, Duration

Pregnancy Related Concerns: Oxymetazoline has the theoretical potential to increase blood pressure and cause a decrease in blood flow to the uterus. This has not been shown to occur in clinical studies of normal pregnancies.

Comments: Follow the manufacturers' recommendations carefully. Use for no more than three days as a bothersome rebound congestion may occur thereafter. Do not use if your baby is growing poorly or you have high blood pressure. A safer decongestant in pregnancy is pseudoephedrine.

Generic Name: PAMABROM
Class of Drug: Diuretic
Use: Reduces fluid retention, increases urine output
Common Brand Names: Aqua-Ban Maximum Strength, Fem-1, Midol Teen Maximum Strength, Midol Maximum Strength PMS, Pamprin, Premsyn, Vitelle Lurline PMS

Pregnancy Related Concerns: Not known to cause malformations, however, very little information is available on this medication. This medicine increases urine output and may be useful uf you have a lot of annoying fluid retention. Unfortunately, it may also be harmful if you have pre-eclampsia. Check with your doctor before using this medicine in the last three months of pregnancy.

Generic Name:	PHENAZOPYRIDINE HYDROCHLORIDE
Class of Drug:	Bladder analgesic
Use:	Relief of symptoms associated with a bladder infection
Common Brand Names:	Azo-100, Azo-Standard, Baridium

Pregnancy Related Concerns: Not known to cause malformations or pregnancy-related problems.

Comments: This medicine does not cure bladder infections and should not be used as a substitute for antibiotics. Urine color and urine tests may be affected by phenazopyridine. If bladder symptoms persist for more than two days, consult with your doctor.

Generic Name:	PHENYLEPHRINE (C)
Class of Drug:	Decongestant
Use:	Relief of nasal and sinus congestion, Hemorrhoid relief (topical)
Common Brand Names*:	Alka-Seltzer Plus Cold, Codimal DM, Preparation H

Pregnancy Related Concerns: Products containing phenylephrine may increase a woman's blood pres-

77

sure as well as decreasing the blood flow to the uterus and the developing baby. The amount absorbed by using this medicine topically for hemorrhoid relief is probably insufficient to be of concern to the developing fetus. Safety in the first 13 weeks of pregnancy is questionable.

Comments: A safer oral decongestant in pregnancy is pseudoephedrine.

Generic Name: **PHENYLTOLOXAMINE**
Class of Drug: Antihistamine
Use: Frequent additive for analgesics and decongestants
Common Brand Names: Aceta-Gesic, FemBack, Flextra-DS, Major-gesic, Percogesic, Phenylgesic

Pregnancy Related Concerns: Very little scientific information is available on this medication.

Comments: Because no useful information is available and other similar medications are more well-studied, it is advisable to use them rather than this one.

Generic Name: **POLYMYXIN b (B)**
Class of Drug: Antibiotic
Use: First aid for cuts, scrapes, burns and skin infections
Common Brand Names*: Betadine First Aid Antibiotics, Neosporin, Polysporin

Pregnancy Related Concerns: Polymyxin b has not been associated with fetal malformations or other pregnancy related problems.

Generic Name: **POVIDONE-IODINE (D)**
Class of Drug: Topical antiseptic
Use: Antiseptic treatment of minor skin injuries.
Common Brand Names: Betadine Antiseptic, Massengill Medicated Douche, Minidyne, Polydine, Summer's Eve Medicated Douche

Pregnancy Related Concerns: The main concern with the use of this product during pregnancy relates to the potential effect of iodide on the fetal thyroid gland. The amount of povidone-iodine absorbed into the maternal circulation when used properly for small cuts and abrasions is extremely small. Therefore, the possibility of damage to the fetal thyroid gland is remote. However, use of this medication in a vaginal douche or on large injuries for several days may potentially result in sufficient maternal absorption to significantly affect fetal thyroid function.

Comments: Use on small cuts and abrasions only. For larger areas of injury or long-term usage needs, it is wiser to use another antibiotic medication. Do not use as a vaginal douche during pregnancy.

Generic Name: **PRAMOXINE HYDROCHLORIDE**
Class of Drug: Topical anesthetic, hemorrhoid care
Use: Relief of minor skin irritations
Common Brand Names*: Caladryl, Procto Foam, Tronolane

Pregnancy Related Concerns: Not known to cause fetal malformations or pregnancy-related problems. However, scientific information is scarce.

Comments: Use according to manufacturers' recommendations.

Generic Name: **PSEUDOEPHEDRINE (C)**
Class of Drug: Decongestant
Use: Relief of nasal and sinus congestion due to colds
Common Brand Names*: Contac, Dristan Cold and Flu, Sudafed

Pregnancy Related Concerns: Unable to be absolutely certain about the safety of any decongestant in the first 13 weeks of pregnancy. After that, sporadic use of this decongestant has not been reported to cause neonatal problems. It has the potential to increase blood pressure in susceptible individuals. Those pregnant women with high blood pressure would be wise to avoid frequent use of these decongestants.

Comments: Of all of the decongestants, pseudoephedrine is most likely the safest.

Generic Name: **PSYLLIUM**
Class of Drug: Laxative--Bulk Agent
Use: Relief of constipation
Common Brand Names*:   Fiberall, Metamucil, Perdiem

Pregnancy Related Concerns: Very little if any of bulk agents is absorbed from the intestinal system. Therefore, the possibility that they could affect a baby is remote.

Comments: Constipation is a very frequent problem in pregnancy. The first step in treating constipation in pregnancy is to increase dietary fiber and fluids. Only if that is unsuccessful should laxative products be considered. Bulking agents are the next logical step for relief of constipation if dietary changes prove unsuccessful. It is important to use this and all laxatives very sporadically and only as needed. Some medications containing bulk agents have a great deal of sugar in them which may increase the blood sugar levels of women who have diabetes during pregnancy.

Generic Name: **PYRETHRINS WITH PIPERONYL BUTOXIDE (C)**

Class of Drug: Pediculocide
Use: Treatment of lice infestation
Common Brand Names: Blue Gel, Clear Total Lice Elimination System, End-Lice, Li Ban, Lice-Enz, Pronto Lice Killing Shampoo, Rid

Pregnancy Related Concerns: This medication is absorbed extremely poorly through the skin so that the potential toxicity for developing babies should be extremely small. For this reason, the use of this medicine is preferred over lindane during pregnancy. It is not effective for the treatment of scabies.

Comments: This is the preferred medicine to use during pregnancy for treatment of lice.

Generic Name: **PYRILAMINE**
Class of Drug: Antihistamine
Use: Combined with decongestants and cough medications, sleep aid
Common Brand Names: Midol Maximum Strength, Pamprin Multi-Symptom Maximum Strength, Premsyn

Pregnancy Related Concerns: Not known to cause fetal malformations. Rarely, premature babies whose mothers have taken antihistamines just prior to premature delivery, have developed an eye disorder (retrolental fibroplasia).

Comments: Avoid daily use in the last thee months of pregnancy if premature labor is a concern.

Generic Name: **PYRITHIONE ZINC**
Class of Drug: Anti-seborrheic
Use: Treatment of dandruff and seborrhea

Common Brand Names: DHS Zinc, Zincon, ZNP Bar

Pregnancy Related Concerns: No known fetal or pregnancy-related concerns if used according to manufacturers' suggestions.

Generic Name: **RANITIDINE (B)**
Class of Drug: Histamine H2-receptor antagonist, antacid
Use: Relief of heartburn
Common Brand Names: Zantac

Pregnancy Related Concerns: Not known to cause malformations. This medication may change the effectiveness of a variety of prescription medications. This concern should be discussed with a physician or pharmacist. When taking certain antacids, the effectiveness of ranitidine is decreased.

Comments: If antacids alone are insufficient for relief of heartburn symptoms, these types of medications often work very well. It works best if taken twice a day. Do not take antacids at the same time. Most pediatricians recommend avoiding use of ranitidine while breastfeeding as it may affect the baby's stomach acid production.

Generic Name: **RESORCINOL**
Class of Drug: Topical anti-infective and antipruritic
Use: Treatment of acne and minor skin irritations

Common Brand Names*:   Bicozene, Resinol, Vagisil

Pregnancy Related Concerns: Not known to cause fetal malformations or pregnancy-related problems
when used according to manufacturers' suggestions.

Generic Name:	**SALICYLATES (C/D)**
Class of Drug:	Analgesic
Use:	Pain relief
Common Brand Names*:	Doan's, Momentum

Pregnancy Related Concerns: Not known to cause malformations.
Use of salicylates may cause tempo-
rary maternal or fetal bleeding problems. Long term use is associated
with prolonged pregnancy and ineffective contractions at the time of
labor.

Comments: Avoid frequent use of this medicine
during pregnancy. Do not use in the
last eight weeks of pregnancy.

Generic Name:	**SALICYLIC ACID**
Class of Drug:	Skin care medication
Use:	Treatment of corns, calluses, warts and other blemishes
Common Brand Names*:	Aveenobar Medicated, Clearasil Clearstick, Compound W

Pregnancy Related Concerns: Although salicylic acid is related
chemically to aspirin, the amount of
medication which would be absorbed
during use of this medicine is

extraordinarily small and unlikely to have any effect on pregnancy when used according to the manufacturers' directions.

Generic Name: **SELENIUM SULFIDE**
Class of Drug: Antiseborrheic
Use: Treatment of dandruff and seborrhea
Common Brand Names: Head and Shoulders, Selsun Blue

Pregnancy Related Concerns: Selenium is poorly absorbed through the skin. Therefore when used according to the manufacturers' suggestions, the potential for affecting a growing baby is remote.

Generic Name: **SENNA AND SENNOSIDES** (C)
Class of Drug: Laxative-stimulant
Use: Relief of constipation
Common Brand Names*:   Ex-Lax, Fletcher's Castoria, Senokot

Pregnancy Related Concerns: Not known to cause fetal malformations. In general, stimulant laxatives are the last resort of treatment for constipation during pregnancy. These should be used rarely. Other methods of constipation relief should be tried first. Dietary changes of increasing fiber and fluid intake, and bulk agent laxatives should be tried prior to using any stimulant laxative. The use of stimulant laxatives will not precipitate labor.

Comments: Avoid stimulant laxatives unless

dietary changes and bulk agent laxatives have failed to result in correction of constipation. Chronic use of stimulant laxatives can result in long-standing or permanent bowel dysfunction.

Generic Name:	**SIMETHICONE (C)**
Class of Drug:	Antiflatulent
Use:	Relief of discomforts of intestinal gas
Common Brand Names:	Anti-Gas, Gas-X, Phazyme

Pregnancy Related Concerns: Not known to cause malformations

Comments: Simethicone is very helpful for many pregnant women who suffer from discomforts from too much gas in their intestinal system. It appears to have no side effects when taken in the proper dosage.

Generic Medication:	**SODIUM BICARBONATE**
Class of Drug:	Antacid
Use:	Relief of heartburn
Common Brand Names*:	Alka-Seltzer, Bromo-Seltzer, Citrocarbonate

Pregnancy Related Concerns: Not known to cause malformations. Sometimes associated with an increase in intestinal gas and stomach distention which is frequently a problem for many pregnant women.

Comments: Not as good for long-term use in pregnancy as other antacids.

Generic Name:	SODIUM SALICYLATE (See Salicylates p. 84)

Generic Name:	SULPHUR
Class of Drug:	Topical keratolytic
Use:	Treatment of dandruff, psoriasis and acne
Common Brand Names*:	Acno, Fostex, Sebulex
Pregnancy Related Concerns:	No known fetal or pregnancy related problems when used according to manufacturers' suggestions.

Generic Name:	TETRAHYDROZOLINE HYDROCHLORIDE
Class of Drug:	Optic decongestant
Use:	Relief of minor eye irritations
Common Brand Names:	Murine Plus, Soothe
Pregnancy Related Concerns:	No known pregnancy related problems when taken according to the manufacturers' suggestions.
Comments:	Do not use this medicine for more than three consecutive days because a rebound worsening of congestion may occur.

Generic Name:	TOLNAFTATE
Class of Drug:	Antifungal agent for skin care use.
Use:	Treatment of minor fungal skin infections
Common Brand Names*:	Absorbine Jr, Tinactin
Pregnancy Related Concerns:	Not known to cause fetal malforma-

tions or other pregnancy related problems when used in the dosage recommended by the manufacturer. The amount of this medicine absorbed into the general circulation after use on skin is extremely small and thus the potential for causing an effect on the baby is remote.

Generic Medication:	**TRIPROLIDINE**
Class of Drug:	Antihistamine
Use:	Relief of allergy symptoms, additive with many decongestants
Common Brand Names*:	Actifed Cold & Allergy, Cenafed

Pregnancy Related Concerns: Not known to cause malformations. Rarely, very premature babies whose mothers who have taken antihistamines just prior to premature delivery have developed an eye disorder (retrolental fibroplasia). This precaution is for all antihistamines.

Comments: Found in a wide variety of combination medications for relief of cold symptoms. Avoid daily use in the last three months of pregnancy if premature labor is a concern.

Generic Name: **TROLAMINE SALICYLATE** (see Salicylates p. 84).

Generic Name:	**UNDECYLENATE SALTS**
Class of Drug:	Topical antifungal agent
Use:	Treatment of minor fungal skin infections

Common Brand Names: Cruex Powder, Desenex, Desenex Maximum Strength, Undelenic Ointment

Pregnancy Related Concerns: Not known to cause fetal malformations or other pregnancy related problems when used in the dosage recommended by the manufacturer. The amount of this medicine absorbed into the general circulation after topical use is extremely small and thus the potential for causing an effect on the baby is remote.

Generic Name:
Class of Drug:
Use:

VITAMINS
Dietary Supplements
Of the many vitamins in a multivitamin capsule, only folic acid has been shown to be of significant benefit in early pregnancy (See p. 58). Most pregnant women can easily consume an adequate supply of the other vitamins by eating a normal diet. The Institute of Medicine does not recommend routine multivitamin supplementation (1990). Taking prenatal multiple vitamins frequently results in unnecessary and undesired nausea, vomiting, bloating, and constipation.

Comments: There are some women who, for a variety of reasons, have inadequate dietary absorption of vitamins and would benefit from a daily multivitamin tablet. Your physician can determine if you require additional vitamins. It is wise to take folic acid prior to and during early pregnancy. However you should take additional multivitamin supplements in early pregnancy only when specifically instructed to do so by your doctor or midwife.

Generic Name:	**ZINC OXIDE**
Class of Drug:	Topical astringent, antiseptic and skin protectant
Use:	Skin protection and relief of minor irritations, hemorrhoid care
Common Brand Names*:	Desitin, Mexana, Wyanoids
Pregnancy Related Concerns:	Zinc oxide does not absorb through the skin, and thus the potential for any effect on the baby is remote.

Index

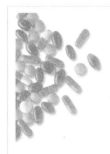

Advantage 24 (See Nonoxynol-9, 75)
Advil (See Ibuprofen, 60)
Advil Flu & Body Ache (See Ibuprofen, 60 and
    Pseudoephedrine, 80)
Aerdil (See Pseudoephedrine, 80 and Triprolidine, 88)
AeroCaine (See Benzocaine, 39)
Aerotherm (See Benzocaine, 39)
Afko-Lube (See Docusate Sodium, 55)
Afko-Lube Lax (See Casanthranol, 46 and Docusate Salts, 55)
Afrin Nasal Spray (See Oxymetazoline Hydrochloride, 76)
Afrinol Repetabs (See Pseudoephedrine, 80)
After Burn (See Lidocaine, 64)
Agoral (See Senna, 85)
Alamag (See Aluminum Hydroxide, 36 and Magnesium Salts, 67)
Alamag Plus (See Aluminum Hydroxide, 36, Magnesium Salts
    p.67 , and Simethicone, 86)
Al-Ay (See Aspirin, 37 , Caffeine, 42 , Chlorpheniramine, 49,
    and Phenylephrine, 77)
Alenic Alka (See Aluminum Hydroxide, 36
    and Magnesium Salts, 77)
Alert-Pep (See Caffeine, 42)
Aleve (See Naproxyn, 72)
Aleve Cold & Sinus (See Naproxyn, 72 and Pseudoephedrine, 80)
Algel (See Aluminum Hydroxide, 36 and Magnesium Salts, 67)
Algenic Alka (See Aluminum Hydroxide, 36 and Magnesium
    Hydroxide, 67)
Algex (See Camphor, 45 , Menthol, 69, and Methylsalicylate, 70)
Alikal (See Sodium Bicarbonate, 86)
Alka-Med Tablets (See Aluminum Hydroxide, 37 and Magnesium
    Salts, 67)
Alka-Mints (See Calcium Carbonate, 44)
Alka-Seltzer (See Aspirin, 37 and Sodium Bicarbonate, 86)
Alka-Seltzer Extra Strength (See Aspirin, 37 and Sodium
    Bicarbonate, 86)
Alka-Seltzer Heartburn Relief (See Sodium Bicarbonate, 86)

Alka-Seltzer Morning Relief (See Aspirin, 37 and Caffeine, 42)

Alka-Seltzer Plus Cold (See Acetaminophen, 35, Chlorpheniramine, 49 and Phenylephrine, 77)

Alka-Seltzer Plus Cold (Liqui-gels) (See Acetaminophen, 35, Chlorpheniramine, 49 and Pseudoephedrine, 80)

Alka-Seltzer Plus Cold & Cough (See Dextromethorphan, 52, Phenylephrine, 77 and Sodium Bicarbonate, 86)

Alka-Seltzer Plus Cold & Cough (Liqui-gels) (See Acetaminophen 35 , Chlorpheniramine, 49, Dextromethorphan, 52, and Pseudoephedrine, 80)

Alka-Seltzer Plus Cold & Sinus (See Acetaminophen, 35, Phenylephrine, 77 and Sodium Bicarbonate, 86)

Alka-Seltzer Plus Cold & Sinus (Liqui-gels) (See Acetaminophen, 35 and Pseudoephedrine, 80)

Alka-Seltzer Plus Flu (See Aspirin, 37, Chlorpheniramine, 49, Dextromethorphan, 52 and Sodium Bicarbonate, 86)

Alka-Seltzer Plus Flu (Liqui-gels) (See Acetaminophen, 35, Dextromethorphan, 52 and Pseudoephedrine, 80)

Alka-Seltzer Plus Night-Time Cold (Liqui-gels) (See Acetaminophen, 35, Dextromethorphan, 52, Doxylamine, 56 and Phenylephrine 77)

Alka-Seltzer Plus Night-Time Cold Medicine (See Dextromethorphan 52, Doxylamine, 56 and Pseudoephedrine, 80)

Alka-Seltzer PM (See Aspirin, 37 and Diphenhydramine, 54)

Alkets (See Calcium Carbonate, 44)

All Clear (See Naphazoline, 71)

Allerest Eye Drops (See Naphazoline, 71)

Allerest Nasal Spray (See Oxymetazoline, 76)

Allerest Maximum Strength (See Chlorpheniramine, 49 and Pseudoephedrine, 80)

Allerest Sinus Pain Formula (See Acetaminophen, 35, Chlorpheniramine, 49 and Pseudoephedrine, 80)

Allerfrim (See Pseudoephedrine, 80 and Triprolidine, 88)

Allergy (See Chlorpheniramine, 49)

AllerMax (See Diphenhydramine, 54)

AllerMax Allergy & Cough Formula (See Diphenhydramine, 54 and Menthol, 69)

Allersone (See Hydrocortisone, 59 and Zinc Oxide, 90)

All-Nite Cold Formula (See Acetaminophen, 35 , Dextromethorphan, 52, Doxylamine, 56, and Pseudoephedrine, 80)

Almacone (See Aluminum Hydroxide, 36, Magnesium Salts, 67, and Simethicone, 86)

Almora (See Magnesium Salts, 67)

Alophen (See Bisacodyl, 40)

Alphaderm (See Hydrocortisone, 59)

Alpha-galactosidase, 36

Alsorb Gel (See Aluminum Hydroxide, 36 and Magnesium Salts, 67)

AlternaGEL (See Aluminum Hydroxide, 36)

Alu-Cap (See Aluminum Hydroxide, 36)

Al-U-Crème (See Aluminum Hydroxide, 36)

Aludrox (See Aluminum Hydroxide, 36 and Magnesium Salts, 67)

Alumate HC (See Hydrocortisone, 59)

Aluminum Hydroxide, 36

Alurex (See Aluminum Hydroxide, 36)

Alu-tab (See Aluminum Hydroxide, 36)

Ambenyl-D (See Dextromethorphan, 52, Guaifenesin, 59 , and Pseudoephedrine, 80)

AMBI 10 Cream (See Benzoyl Peroxide, 39)

Americaine (See Benzocaine, 39)

Americaine Hemorrhoidal (See Benzocaine, 39)

Aminofen (See Acetaminophen, 35)

Amitone (See Calcium Carbonate, 44)

Ammens (See Zinc Oxide, 90)

Amphojel (See Aluminum Hydroxide, 36)

Anacaine (See Benzocaine, 39)

Anacin (See Aspirin, 37, and Caffeine, 42)

Anacin Aspirin Free Maximum-Strength (See Acetaminophen, 35)

Analbalm Improved Formula (See Menthol, 59 and Methyl Salicylate, 70)

Anatuss DM (See Dextromethorphan, 52, Guaifenesin, 59 and
    Pseudoephedrine, 80)
Anbesol (See Benzocaine, 39)
Anodynos (See Aspirin, 37, Caffeine, 42 and Salicylates, 84)
Antacid Extra Strength (See Calcium Carbonate, 44)
Antacid Suspension (See Aluminum Hydroxide 36, and
    Magnesium Salts, 67)
Anti-Gas (See Simethicone, 86)
Anti-Itch (See Pramoxine, 80)
Anti-Tuss (See Guaifenesin, 59)
Anti-Tuss DM (See Dextromethorphan, 52 and Guaifenesin, 59)
Anusol HC (See Hydrocortisone, 59)
Anusol Ointment (See Pramoxine, 80 and Zinc Oxide, 90)
Apap (See Acetaminophen, 35)
Apap Plus (See Acetaminophen, 35 and Caffeine, 42)
A.P.C. (See Aspirin, 37 and Caffeine, 42)
Aprodine (See Pseudoephedrine, 80 and Triprolidine, 88)
Aqua-Ban, Maximum Strength (See Pamabrom, 76)
Arcodex (See Aluminum Hydroxide, 36 and Magnesium Salts, 67)
Arthricare Double Ice (See Camphor, 45)
Arthritic Pain (See Salicylates, 84)
Arthritis Hot Crème (See Salicylates, 84 and Menthol, 69)
Arthritis Foundation Aspirin Free (See Acetaminophen, 35)
Arthritis Pain Formula (See Aluminum Hydroxide, 36, Aspirin 37,
    and Magnesium Salts, 67)
A.S.A. (See Aspirin, 37)
Ascriptin (See Aspirin, 37, Aluminum Hydroxide, 36, and
    Magnesium Salts, 67)
Aspercreme (See Salicylates, 84)
Aspergum (See Aspirin, 37)
Aspermin (See Aspirin, 37 and Caffeine, 42)
Aspirin, 37
Aspirin Free Pain Relief (See Acetaminophen, 35)
Aspirtab (See Aspirin, 37)
Asprimox (See Aspirin, 37)

AsthmaNephrin (See Epinephrine, 57)
Asupirin (See Aspirin, 37)
Atridine (See Pseudoephedrine, 80 and Triprolidine, 88)
Atrocholin (See Dehydrocholic Acid, 52)
Attapulgite, 38
Aveeno Anti-Itch (See Calamine, 43, Camphor, 45 and
    Pramoxine, 80)
Aveenobar Medicated (See Salicylic Acid, 84)
Axid (See Nizatidine, 74)
Azo-100 (See Phenazopyridine Hydrochloride, 77)
Azo-Standard (See Phenazopyridine Hydrochloride, 77)

Baciguent (See Bacitracin, 38)
Bacitracin, 38
Backache (See Salicylates, 84)
Bactine First Aid Antibiotic (See Bacitracin, 38, Neomycin, 73,
    and Polymixin, 78)
Bactine Hydrocortisone (See Hydrocortisone, 39)
Balmex (See Zinc Oxide, 90)
Balnetar (See Coal Tar, 52)
Banacid (See Magnesium Salts, 67)
Banalg (See Camphor, 45)
BanSmoke (See Benzocaine, 39)
Band-Aid Plus (See Bacitracin, 39, Neomycin, 73, Polymixin b 78,
    and Pramoxine, 80)
Banophen (See Diphenhydramine, 54)
Baridium (See Phenazopyridine Hydrochloride, 77)
Basa (See Aspirin, 37)
Bayer (See Aspirin, 37)
Bayer Aspirin Arthritis Pain Extra Strength (See Aspirin, 37)
Bayer Plus Extra Strength (See Aspirin, 37)
Bayer PM Extra strength (See Aspirin and Diphenhydramine, 54)
Bayer Select Aspirin Free (See Actaminophen, 35)

Bayer Women's Aspirin Plus Calcium (See Aspirin, 37 and Calcium, 43)

BC Allergy Sinus Cold Powder (See Aspirin, 37, Chlorpheniramine, 49, and Pseudoephedrine, 80)

BC Arthritis Strength (See Aspirin, 37 and Caffeine, 42)

BC Sinus Cold Powder (See Aspirin, 37 and Pseodoephedrine, 80)

BC Powder (See Aspirin, 37, and Caffeine, 42)

Beano (See Alpha-galactosidase, 36)

Beldin (See Diphenhydramine, 54)

Bell/ans (See Sodium Bicarbonate, 86)

Benadryl (See Diphenhydramine, 54)

Benadryl Allergy & Cold (See Acetaminophen, 35, Diphenhydramine, 54 and Pseudoephedrine, 80)

Benadryl Allergy & Sinus (See Diphenhydramine, 54 and Pseudoephedrine, 80)

Benadryl Allergy & Sinus Headache (See Acetaminophen, 35, Diphenhydramine, 54, and Pseudoephedrine, 80)

Benadryl Maximum Strength Severe Allergy & Sinus Headache (See Acetaminophen, 35 , Diphenhydramine, 54 and Pseudoephedrine, 80)

Ben-Gay Extra Strength (See Menthol, 69 and Methyl Salicylate, 70)

Ben-Gay SPA (See Menthol, 69)

Ben-Gay Sportsgel (See Menthol, 69 and Methyl Salicylate, 70)

Benoxyl (See Benzoyl Peroxide, 39)

Bensulfoid (See Resorcinol, 83 and Sulphur, 87)

Benylin Adult Cough Formula (See Dextromethorphan, 52)

Benylin DM (See Dextromethorphan, 52)

Benylin Expectorant (See Dextromethorphan, 52 and Guaifenesin, 59)

Benylin Multi-Symptom Formula (See Dextromethorphan, 52, Guaifenesin, 59 and Pseudoephedrine, 80)

Benzo-C (See Benzocaine, 39)

Benzocaine, 39

Benzodent (See Benzocaine, 39)

Benzoyl Peroxide, 39

Betadine Antiseptic (See Povidone-Iodine, 79)

Betadine Cream (See Povidone-Iodine, 79)
Betadine First Aid Antibiotics (See Bacitracin, 38 and Polymyxin, 78)
Betadine Medicated Douche (See Povidone-Iodine, 79)
Betadine Medicated Vaginal Gel and Suppositories
    (See Povidone-Iodine, 79)
Betadine PrepStick (See Povidone-Iodine, 79)
Betadine Shampoo (See Povidone-Iodine, 79)
Bicozene (See Benzocaine, 39)
B-K-P (See Kaolin, 62)
Bilax (See Dehydrocholic acid, 52)
Bilstan (See Cascara, 47)
Biocal 250, 500 (See Calcium, 43)
Bisac-Evac (See Bisacodyl, 40)
Bisacodyl, 40
Bismuth Subsalicylate, 40
Black and White Ointment (See Resorcinol, 83)
Black-Draught (See Senna, 85)
Blaud Strubel (See Iron, 61)
Blis-To-Sol (Liquid) (See Tolnaftate, 87)
Blue (See Pyrethrins with Piperonyl Butoxide, 81)
Blue Gel Muscular Pain Relief (See Menthol, 69)
Blue Star (See Camphor, 45)
Boil Ease (See Benzocaine, 39)
Bonine (See Meclizine, 68)
Borofax Skin Protectant (See Zinc Oxide, 90)
Breezee-Mist Antifungal (See Miconazole, 70)
Brexin (See Pseudoephedrine, 80)
Brexin-EX (See Guaifenesin, 59 and Pseudoephedrine, 80)
Bromanate (See Brompheniramine, 41 and Pseudoephedrine, 80)
Bromatap (See Brompheniramine, 41 and Phenylephrine, 77)
Bromfed (See Brompheniramine, 41 and Pseudoephedrine, 80)
Bromfed-DM (See Brompheniramine, 41, Dextromethorphan 52,
    and Pseudoephedrine, 80)
Bromo-Seltzer (See Acetaminophen, 35 and Sodium Bicarbonate, 86)
Brompheniramine, 41

Bronitin (See Ephedrine, 56, Guaifenesin, 59 and Pyrilamine, 82)
Bronitin Mist (See Epinephrine, 57)
Bronkaid Dual Action (See Ephedrine, 56 and Guaifenesin, 59)
Buf-Bar (See Sulphur, 87)
Buff-A (See Aspirin, 37 and Magnesium Salts, 67)
Buffaprin (See Aspirin, 37)
Bufferin (See Aspirin, 37)
Bufferin AF Nite Time (See Acetaminophen, 35 and
    Diphenhydramine, 54)
Buffex (See Aspirin, 37)
Buf-Puf Medicated (See Salicylic Acid, 84)
Bulk Forming Fiber Laxative (See Calcium Polycarbophil, 45)
Butoconazole, 41
Bydramine (See Diphenhydramine, 54)

Caffedrine (See Caffeine, 42)
Caffeine, 42
Caladryl (See Camphor, 45, Calamine, 43 and Pramoxine, 80)
Calahist (See Calamine, 43 and Diphenhydramine, 54)
Calamatum (See Benzocaine, 39, Calamine, 43 and Zinc Oxide, 90)
Calamine, 43
Calamox (See Calamine, 43)
Calamycin (See Calamine, 43, Pramoxine , 80 and Zinc Oxide, 90)
Cal-Carb Forte (See Calcium, 43)
Calcet (See Calcium, 43)
Calci-Chew (See Calcium, 43)
Calci-Mix (See Calcium, 43)
Cal-Citrate (See Calcium, 43)
Calcium, 43
Calcium 600 (See Calcium, 43)
Calcium Carbimide, 44
Calcium Carbonate, 44
Calcium Polycarbophil, 45

CaldeCORT (See Hydrocortisone, 59)
Caldesene Medicated Ointment (See Zinc Oxide, 90)
Calicylic (See Salicylic Acid, 84)
Cal-Lac (See Calcium, 43)
Calmol 4 (See Zinc Oxide, 90)
Calotabs (See Casanthranol, 46)
Caltrate 600 (See Calcium, 43)
Caltro (See Calcium, 43)
Cama (See Aluminum Hydroxide, 36 and Aspirin, 37)
Campho-Phenique (See Camphor, 45)
Camphor, 45
Ca-Orotate (See Calcium, 43)
Capsaicin, 46
Capsin (See Capsaicin, 46)
Capzasin-P (See Capsaicin, 46)
Carter's Little Pills (See Bisacodyl, 40)
Casanthranol, 46
Cascara, 47
Cascara Aromatic (See Cascara, 47)
Castor Oil, 48
Cenafed Plus (See Pseudoephedrine, 80 and Triprolidine, 88)
Cenafed Syrup (See Pseudoephedrine, 80)
Cenafed Tablets (See Pseudoephedrine, 80)
Cepacol Anesthetic Lozenges (See Benzocaine, 39)
Cepacol Maximum Strength (See Benzocaine, 39)
Cepacol Sore Throat (See Acetaminophen, 35 and
    Pseudoephedrine, 80)
Ceretex (See Iron, 61)
Cerose (See Chlorpheniramine, 49, Dextromethorphan, 52 and
    Phenylephrine, 77)
CharcoAid (See Charcoal, 48)
Charcoal, 48
Charcoal Plus (See Charcoal, 48)
CharcoCaps (See Charcoal, 48)
Charo Scatter-Paks (See Charcoal, 48)

Cheracol D (See Dextromethorphan, 52 and Guaifenesin, 59)
Cheracol Plus (See Dextromethorphan, 52 and Guaifenesin, 59)
Cheratussin Cough (See Dextromethorphan, 52)
Chiggerex (See Benzocaine, 39 and Camphor, 45)
Chigger-Tox (See Benzocaine, 39)
Childron (See Iron, 61)
Chlo-Amine (See Chlorpheniramine, 49)
Chloren (See Chlorpheniramine, 49)
Chlor-Niramine Allergy Tabs (See Chlorpheniramine, 49)
Chlorphed-LA (See Oxymetazoline Hydrochloride, 76)
Chlorpheniramine, 49
Chlor-Span (See Chlorpheniramine, 49)
Chlor-Trimeton Allergy Tablets (See Chlorpheniramine, 49)
Chlor-Trimeton Allergy/Decongestant Tablets
    (See Chlorpheniramine, 49 and Pseudoephedrine, 80)
Chlor-Trimeton 12 Hour Relief (See Chlorpheniramine, 49
    and Pseudoephedrine, 80)
Cholan DH (See Dehydrocholic Acid, 52)
Chooz (See Calcium carbonate, 44)
Cimetidine, 49
Citracal (See Calcium, 43)
Citra Forte (See Phenylephrine, 77)
Citrocarbonate (See Sodium Bicarbonate, 86)
Citroma (See Magnesium Salts, 67)
Citrucel (See Methylcellulose, 69)
Citrucel Sugar Free (See Methylcellulose, 69)
Claritin (See Loratadine, 66)
Clean and Clear Invisible Blemish Treatment (See Salicylic Acid, 84)
Clean and Clear Oil Controlling Astringent (See Salicylic Acid, 84)
Clearasil Adult Care Cream (See Resorcinol, 83)
Clearasil Clearstick (See Salicylic Acid, 84)
Clearasil Maximum Strength Cream (See Benzoyl Peroxide, 39)
Clearasil 10% (See Benzoyl Peroxide, 39)
Clear Away One-Step Wart Remover (See Salicylic Acid, 84)
Clear Away Plantar Wart Remover (See Salicylic Acid, 84)

Clear Cough DM (See Dextromethorphan, 52 and Guaifenesin, 59)

Clear Eyes (Naphazoline Hydrochloride, 71)

Clear Total Lice Elimination System (See Pyrethrins with Piperonyl Butoxide, 81)

Clear Tussin 30 (See Dextromethorphan, 52 and Guaifenesin, 59)

Clemastine, 50

Clinac (See Benzoyl Peroxide, 39)

Clorfed II (See Chlorpheniramine, 49 and Pseudoephedrine, 80)

Clotrimazole, 51

Coadvil (See Ibuprofen, 60 and Pseudoephedrine, 80)

Coal Tar, 52

Co-Apap (See Acetaminophen, 35, Chlorpheniramine, 49, Dextromethorphan, 52 and Pseudoephedrine, 80)

Codimal (See Acetaminophen, 35, Chlorpheniramine, 49 and Pseudoephedrine, 80)

Codimal DM (See Dextromethorphan, 52 and Phenylephrine, 77)

Co-Hist (See Acetaminophen, 35, Chlorpheniramine, 49 and Pseudoephedrine, 80)

Colace (See Docusate Salts, 55)

Coldrine (See Acetaminophen, 35 and Pseudoephedrine, 80)

Cold-Gest Cold (See Chlorpheniramine, 49 and Pseudoephedrine, 80)

Comfort Eye Drops (See Naphazoline Hydrochloride, 71)

Comfort Gel Liquid (See Aluminum Hydroxide, 36 and Magnesium Salts, 67)

Comfort Gel Tablets (See Magnesium Salts, 67 and Simethicone, 86)

Completone Elixir Fort (See Iron, 61)

Compound W Wart Remover (See Salicylic Acid, 84)

Compoz (See Diphenhydramine, 54)

Comtrex (See Acetaminophen, 35, Chlorpheniramine, 49, Dextromethorphan, 52 and Pseudoephedrine, 80)

Comtrex Maximum Strength Acute Head Cold Caplets (See Acetaminophen, 35, Brompheniramine, 41 and Pseudoephedrine, 80)

Comtrex Maximum Strength Cold & Cough Day & Night Caplets (See Acetaminophen, 35, Dextromethorphan, 52 and

Pseudeophedrine, 80)

Comtrex Maximum Strength Flu Therapy Day & Night
  (See Acetaminophen, 35, Chlorpheniramine, 49, and
  Pseudeophedrine, 80)

Comtrex Maximum Strength Sinus & Nasal Congestion
  (See Acetaminophen, 35, Chlorpheniramine, 49 and
  Pseudoephedrine, 80)

Comtrex Multi-Symptom Deep Chest Cold (See Acetaminophen 35,
  Dextromethorphan, 52, Guaifenesin, 59 and Pseudoephedrine, 80)

Concentrin (See Dextromethorphan, 52, Guaifenesin, 59 and
  Pseudoephedrine, 80)

Conceptrol (See Nonoxynol-9, 75)

Congestac (See Guaifenesin, 59 and Pseudoephedrine, 80)

Contac Non-Drowsy Decongestant 12 Hour Cold Caplets
  (See Pseudoephedrine, 80)

Contac Non-Drowsy Timed Release 12 Hour Cold Caplets
  (See Pseudoephedrine, 80)

Contac Severe Cold & Flu Maximum Strength (See Acetaminophen
  35, Dextromethorphan, 52 and Pseudoephedrine, 80)

Contac Severe Cold & Flu Non- Drowsy (See Acetaminophen, 35,
  Dextromethorphan, 52 and Pseudoephedrine, 80)

Cope (See Aluminum Hydroxide, 36, Aspirin, 37, Caffeine, 42,
  and Magnesium Hydroxide, 67)

Coricidin HBP Cold & Flu (See Acetaminophen, 35 and
  Chlorpheniramine, 49)

Coricidin HBP Cough & Cold (See Chlorpheniramine, 49 and
  Dextromethorphan, 52)

Coricidin HBP Maximum Strength Flu Tablets
  (See Acetaminophen, 35, Chlorpheniramine, 49 and
  Dextromethorphan, 52)

Coricin "D" Cold Flu & Sinus (See Acetaminophen, 35,
  Chlorpheniramine, 49 and Pseudoephedrine, 80)

Corn Fix (See Salicylic Acid, 84)

Correctol (See Bisacodyl, 40)

Correctol Extra Gentle (See Docusate Salts, 55)

Cortaid (See Hydrocortisone, 59)
Corticaine Maximum Strength (See Hydrocortisone, 59)
Cortizone-5 (See Hydrocortisone, 59)
Cortizone-10 (See Hydrocortisone, 59)
Coryza Brengle (See Acetaminophen, 35 and Pseudoephedrine, 80)
Co-Tylenol Cold Formula (See Acetaminophen, 35,
    Chlorpheniramine, 49, Dextromethorphan, 52 and
    Pseudoephedrine, 80)
Cough Syrup (See Dextromethorphan, 52, Guaifenesin, 49 and
    Pseudoephedrine, 80)
Cough-X (See Benzocaine, 39 and Dextromethorphan, 52)
Creamy Tar (See Coal Tar, 52)
Creomulsion Cough (See Cascara, 47 and Menthol, 69)
C-Ron (See Iron, 61)
Cruex Powder (See Undecylenate Salts, 88)
Culminal (See Benzocaine, 39)
Cystex (See Salicylates, 84)
Cytoferin (See Iron, 61)

Dacodyl (See Bisacodyl, 40)
DairyEase (See Lactase, 63)
Dapa (See Acetaminophen, 35)
DayHist-1 (See Clemastine, 50)
D-Cal (See Calcium Carbonate, 44)
DC Softgels (See Docusate Salts, 55)
Decapryn (See Doxylamine, 56)
Decholin (See Dehydrocholic Acid, 52)
Decodult (See Acetaminophen, 35, Chlorpheniramine, 49 and
    Phenylephrine, 77)
Decohistine (See Chlorpheniramine, 49 and Phenylephrine, 77)
Deep-Down (See Camphor, 45, Menthol, 69 and Salicylates, 84)
Deficol (See Bisacodyl, 40)
Degest-2 (See Naphazoline Hydrochloride, 71)

Dehydrocholic Acid, 52

Delacort (See Hydrocortisone, 59)

Delcid (See Aluminum Hydroxide, 36 and Magnesium Salts, 67)

Delco-Lax (See Bisacodyl, 40)

Delfen (See Nonoxynol-9, 75)

Delsym (See Dextromethorphan, 52)

Dencorub (See Camphor, 45, Menthol, 69 and Salicylates, 84)

Dencorub Analgesic Liquid (See Capsaicin, 46)

Denorex (See Coal Tar, 52)

Dent's (See Benzocaine, 39)

Dermaflex (See Lidocaine, 64)

Dermamycin (See Diphenhydramine, 54)

Dermarest (See Diphenhydramine, 54)

Dermarest DriCort (See Hydrocortisone, 59)

Dermolate (See Hydrocortisone, 59)

Dermoplast (See Benzocaine, 39)

Desenex (See Undecylenate Salts, 88)

Desenex AF (See Miconazole, 70)

Desenex Cream (See Miconazole, 70)

Desenex Maximum Strength (See Undecylenate Salts, 88)

Desitin (See Zinc Oxide, 90)

Detane (See Benzocaine, 39)

Dexafed (See Dextromethorphan, 52, Guaifenesin, 59, and
    Phenylephrine, 77)

DexAlone (See Dextromethorphan, 52)

Dexitac (See Caffeine, 42)

Dextromethorphan, 52

DHS Zinc (See Pyrithione Zinc, 82)

Diabetic Tussin (See Dextromethorphan, 52 and Guaifenesin, 59)

Diabetic Tussin DM (See Dextromethorphan, 52 and Guaifenesin, 59)

Diabetic Tussin EX (See Guaifenesin, 59 and Menthol, 69)

Diabetic Tussin Maximum Strength (See Dextromethorphan, 52
    and Guaifenesin, 59)

Dialose Plus (See Casanthranol, 46)

Diaperene (See Zinc Oxide, 90)

Diaper Guard (See Zinc Oxide, 90)
Diaper Rash Ointment (See Zinc Oxide, 90)
Diasorb (See Attapulgite, 38)
Diastop (See Kaolin, 62)
Dibucaine, 53
Dicarbosil (See Calcium Carbonate, 44)
Di-Gel (See Aluminum Hydroxide, 36, Magnesium Hydroxide 67, and Simethicone, 86)
Dimacol (See Dextromethorphan, 52, Guaifenesin, 59 and Pseudoephedrine, 80)
Dimaphen (See Brompheniramine, 41 and Pseudoephedrine, 80)
Dimenest (See Dimenhydrinate, 53)
Dimenhydrinate, 53
Dimentabs (See Dimenhydrinate, 53)
Dimetane (See Brompheniramine, 41 and Phenylephrine, 77)
Dimetapp (See Brompheniramine, 41)
Dimetapp DM Cold and Cough (See Brompheniramine, 41, Dextromethorphan, 52 and Pseudoephedrine, 80)
Dimetapp Nighttime Flu Syrup (See Brompheniramine, 41, Dextromethorphan, 52 and Psedoephedrine, 80)
Dimetapp Non-Drowsy Flu Syrup (See Acetaminophen, 35, Dextromethorphan, 52 and Pseudoephedrine, 80)
Dinate (See Dimenhydrinate, 53)
Dioctolose (See Docusate Salts, 55)
Diosate (See Docusate Salts, 55)
Dio-Soft (See Casanthranol, 46)
Diphen (See Diphenhydramine, 54)
Diphenhist (See Diphenhydramine, 54)
Diphenhydramine, 54
Dizmiss (see Meclizine, 68)
DM Cough (See Dextromethorphan, 52)
Doak Tar (See Coal Tar, 52)
Doan's (See Salicylates, 84)
Doctar (See Coal Tar, 52)
Docu (See Docusate Salts, 55)

Docusate Salts, 55
Dolono (See Acetaminophen, 35)
Dolorac (See Capsaicin, 46)
Dorcol (See Acetaminophen, 35)
Dormin (See Diphenhydramine, 54)
D.O.S. (See Docusate Salts, 55)
Dosaflex (See Senna, 85)
Doss (See Docusate Salts, 55)
Double Antibiotic (See Bacitracin, 38 and Polymixin b, 78)
Double Sal (See Salicylates, 84)
Doxidan (See Casanthranol, 46 and Docusate Salts, 55)
Doxylamine, 56
Dramamine (See Dimenhydrinate, 53)
Dramamine Less Drowsy Formula (See Meclizine, 68)
Dramamine II (See Meclizine, 68)
Dramanate (See Dimenhydrinate, 53)
Dr. Dermi-Heal (See Zinc Oxide, 90)
Dr. Drake's Cough Medicine (See Dextromethorphan, 52)
Dristan Allergy (See Brompheniramine, 41 and Pseudoephedrine, 80)
Dristan Cold (See Acetaminophen, 35 and Pseudoephedrine, 80)
Dristan Cold and Flu (See Acetamoniphen, 35, Chlorpheniramine,
     49, Dextromethorphan, 52, and Pseudoephedrine, 80)
Dristan Maximum Strength (See Acetaminophen, 35 and
     Pseudoephedrine, 80)
Dristan Nasal Mist (See Phenylephrine, 77)
Dristan No Drowsiness Cold (See Acetaminophen, 35 and
     Pseudoephedrine, 80)
Dristan Sinus (See Ibuprofen, 60 and Pseudoephedrine, 80)
Dristan 12-Hour Nasal Spray (See Oxymetazoline, 76)
Drixoral Allergy Sinus Extended Relief (See Acetaminophen, 35,
     Brompheniramine, 41, and Pseudoephedrine, 80)
Drixoral Cold and Allergy Sustained Action
     (See Brompheniramine, 41 and Pseudoephedrine, 80)
Drixoral Cold and Flu (See Acetaminophen, 35,
     Brompheniramine, 41 and Pseudoephedrine, 80)

Drixoral Nasal Decongestant (See Pseudoephedrine, 80)
Dr. Scholl's (See Salicylic Acid, 84)
Dr. Scholl's Athlete's Foot (See Tolnaftate, 87)
Drucon (See Chlorpheniramine, 49 and Phenylephrine, 77)
Dryox (See Benzoyl Peroxide, 39)
Dryphen Multi-Symptom (See Acetaminophen, 35,
     Chlorpheniramine, 49 and Phenylephrine, 77)
Drytex (See Salicylic Acid, 84)
DSS (See Docusate Salts, 55)
DSS 100 Plus (See Casanthranol, 46 and Docusate Salts, 55)
Dulcagen (See Bisacodyl, 40)
Dulcolax (See Bisacodyl, 40)
DulFilm Liquid Wart Remover (See Salicylic Acid, 84)
DuoPlant Plantar Wart Remover (See Salicylic Acid, 84)
Duramist Plus 12 Hour Decongestant (See Oxymetazoline
     Hydrochloride, 76)
Duration Nasal Spray (See Oxymetazoline Hydrochloride, 76)
DX 114 Foot Powder (See Salicylic Acid, 84 and Undecylenic Salts, 88)
Dynafed Asthmatic Relief (See Ephedrine, 56 and Guaifenesin, 59)
Dynafed E.X. Extra Strength (See Acetaminophen, 35)
Dyprotex (see Zinc Oxide, 90)

Easprin (See Aspirin, 37)
Easy-Lax (See Docusate Salts, 55)
Easy-Lax Plus (See Casanthranol, 46 and Docusate Salts, 55)
Ecotrin (See Aspirin, 37)
Efedron Nasal (See Ephedrine, 56 and Menthol, 69)
Effective Strength Cough w/Decongestant (See Dextromethorphan,
     52 and Pseudoephedrine, 80)
Effidac 24 (See Chlorpheniramine, 49)
ELA-Max (See Lidocaine, 64)
Eldofe (See Iron, 61)
Emdol (See Salicylates, 84)

Emko (See Nonoxynol-9, 75)
Empirin (See Aspirin, 37)
Emulsoil (See Castor Oil, 48)
Encare (See Nonoxynol-9, 75)
End-Lice (See Pyrethrins with Piperonyl Butoxide, 81)
Enerjets (See Caffeine, 42)
Ephedrine, 56
Epi-Derm Balm (See See Salicylates, 84 and Menthol, 69)
Epinephrine, 56
Epinephrine Mist (See Epinephrine, 56)
Equalactin (See Calcium Polycarbophil, 45)
Estar (See Coal Tar, 52)
Eucalyptamint Maximum Strength (See Menthol, 69)
Evactol (See Docusate Salts, 55)
Eviron (See Iron, 61)
ExACT (See Benzoyl Peroxide, 39)
ExACT Pore Treatment (See Salicylic Acid, 84)
Excedrin Aspirin Free (See Acetaminophen, 35 and Caffeine, 42)
Excedrin Extra-Strength (See Acetaminophen, 35, Aspirin, 37,
    and Caffeine, 42)
Excedrin IB (See Ibuprofen, 60)
Excedrin PM (See Acetaminophen, 35 and Diphenhydramine, 54)
Excedrin Sinus (See Acetaminophen, 35 and Pseudoephedrine, 80)
ex-lax (See Senna, 85)
ex-lax Chocolated (See Senna, 85)
ex-lax Gentle Strength (See Docusate Salts, 55 and Senna, 85)
Extra Action Cough
    (See Dextromethorphan, 52 and Guaifenesin, 59)
Extreme Cold Formula (See Acetaminophen, 35, Chlorpheniramine,
    49, Dextromethorphan, 52 and Pseudoephedrine, 80)

Famotidine, 57
Farbegen (See Iron, 61)

Fastiene (See Caffeine, 42)

Father John's Medicine Plus (See Chlorpheniramine, 49, Dextromethorphan, 52 and Phenylephrine, 77)

F.C.A.H. (See Acetaminophen, 35 and Chlorpheniramine, 49)

Feco-T (See Iron, 61)

Fedahist Expectorant
(See Guaifenesin, 59 and Pseudoephedrine, 80)

Feen-A-Mint (See Bisacodyl, 40)

Feg-1 (See Iron, 61)

FemBack (See Acetaminophen, 35, Phenyltoloxamine 78, and Salicylates, 84)

Fem-Iron (See Iron, 61)

Femizole-M (See Miconazole, 70)

Fem-1 (see Acetaminophen, and Pamabrom, 76)

Femstat-3 (See Butoconazole, 41)

Fendol (See Acetaminophen, 35, Caffeine, 42 and Phenylephrine, 77)

Fenylhist (See Diphenhydramine, 54)

Feosol (See Iron, 61)

Feostat (See Iron, 61)

Ferancee (See Iron, 61)

Feratab (See Iron, 61)

Fer-gen-sol (See Iron, 61)

Fergon (See Iron, 61)

Fer-In-Sol (See Iron, 61)

Fer-Iron (See Iron, 61)

Fero-Folic 500 (See Iron, 61)

Fero-Gradumet (See Iron, 61)

Ferolix (See Iron, 61)

Ferospace (See Iron, 61)

Fer-Regules (See Docusate Salts, 55 and Iron, 61)

Ferretts (See Iron, 61)

Ferro-Docusate (See Docusate Salts, 55 and Iron, 61)

Ferro-Dok (See Docusate Salts, 55 and Iron, 61)

Ferro-DSS SR (See Docusate Salts, 55 and Iron, 61)

Ferrodyl (See Iron, 61)

Ferromar (See Iron, 61)
Ferro-Sequels (See Docusate Salts, 55 and Iron, 61)
Ferrospan (See Iron, 61)
Ferrous Fumarate (See Iron, 61)
Ferrous Gluconate (See Iron, 61)
Ferrous Sulfate (See Iron, 61)
Fesotyme (See Iron, 61)
Feverall (See Acetaminophen, 35)
Fiberall (See Psyllium, 81)
FiberCon (See Calcium Polycarbophil, 45)
FiberNorm (See Calcium Polycarbophil, 45)
First Aid Cream (See Benzocaine, 39)
Flanders Buttocks (See Zinc Oxide, 90)
Flatulex (See Charcoal, 52 and Simethicone, 86)
Fleet Laxative (See Bisacodyl, 40)
Fleet Pain-Relief (See Pramoxine, 80)
Fletcher's Castoria (See Senna, 85)
Flextra-DS (See Acetaminophen, 35 and Phenyltoloxamine, 78)
Florical (See Calcium, 43)
FoilleCort (See Hydrocortisone, 59)
Folic acid, 58
Folvron (See Iron, 61)
Fostex Medicated (See Salicylic Acid, 84)
Fostex 10% (See Benzoyl Peroxide, 39)
Fostril (See Sulphur, 87)
Fumasorb (See Iron, 61)
Fumerin (See Iron, 61)
Fung-O (See Salicylic Acid, 84)
Fungoid Tincture (See Miconazole, 70)

Gacid (See Aluminum Hydroxide, 36 and Magnesium Salts, 67)
Gas Ban (See Calcium Carbonate, 44 and Simethicone, 86)
Gas Ban DS (See Aluminum Hydroxide, 36, Magnesium Salts 67,

and Simethicone, 86)

Gas Relief (See Simethicone, 86)

Gas-X (See Simethicone, 86)

Gaviscon (See Aluminum Hydroxide, 36 and Magnesium Salts, 67)

Gee-Gee (See Guaifenesin, 59)

Gelamal (See Magaldrate, 66)

Genac (See Pseudoephedrine, 80 and Triprolidine, 88)

Genacol Maximum Strength Cold & Flu Relief (See Acetaminophen 35, Chlorpheniramine, 49, Dextromethorphan, 52 and Pseudoephedrine, 80)

Genahist (See Diphenhydramine, 54)

Genapap (See Acetaminophen, 35)

Genaphed (See Pseudoephedrine, 80)

Genasoft (See Docusate Salts, 55)

Genasoft Plus (See Casanthranol, 46 and Docusate Salts, 55)

Genaspor (See Tolnaftate, 87)

Genasyme (See Simethicone, 86)

Genaton (See Aluminum Hydroxide, 36 and Magnesium Salts, 67)

Genatuss DM (See Dextromethorphan, 52 and Guaifenesin, 59)

Genatuss Syrup (See Guaifenesin, 59)

Gendecon (See Acetaminophen, 35, Chlorpheniramine, 49 and Phenylephrine, 77)

Genebs (See Acetaminophen, 35)

Geneye (See Tetrahydrozoline, 87)

Genfiber (See Psyllium, 81)

Genite (See Acetaminophen, 35, Dextromethorphan, 52, Doxylamine, 56, and Pseudoephedrine, 80)

Genna (See Senna, 85)

Genpril (See Ibuprofen, 60)

Genprin (See Aspirin, 37)

Gentle Nature Natural Vegetable Laxatives (See Senna, 85)

Gentz Rectal Wipes (See Pramoxine, 80)

Geritol Tonic Liquid (See Iron, 61)

Ger-O-Foam (See Benzocaine, 39 and Methyl Salicylate, 70)

Glucovite (See Iron, 61)

Glyate (See Guaifenesin, 59)

Glycate Chewables (See Calcium Carbonate, 44)

Glycofed (See Guaifenesin, 59 and Pseudoephedrine, 80)

Glycotuss (See Guaifenesin, 59)

Glycotuss-dM (See Dextromethorphan, 52 and Guaifenesin, 59)

Glytuss (See Guaifenesin, 59)

Gold Seal Calcium 600 (See Calcium, 43)

Gold Seal Ferrous Gluconate (See Iron, 61)

Good Sense Maximum Strength Dose Sinus (See Acetaminophen, 35, Chlorpheniramine, 49 and Pseudoephedrine, 80)

Goody's Body Pain Powder (See Acetaminophen, 35 and Aspirin, 37)

Goody's Headache Powders (See Acetaminophen, 35, Aspirin 37, and Caffeine, 42)

Gordofilm (See Salicylic Acid, 84)

Guaifed Syrup (See Guaifenesin, 59 and Pseudoephedrine, 80)

Guaifenesin, 59

Guaifenesin DM (See Dextromethorphan, 52 and Guaifenesin, 59)

Guaitab (See Pseudoephedrine, 80 and Guaifenesin, 59)

Guiatuss (See Guaifenesin, 59)

Guiatuss CF (See Dextromethorphan, 52, Guaifenesin, 59 and Pseudoephedrine, 80)

Guiatuss PE (See Guaifenesin, 59 and Pseudoephedrine, 80)

Gyne-Lotrimin (See Clotrimazole, 51)

Gynol II (See Nonoxynol-9, 75)

Habitrol (See Nicotine, 74)

Halenol (See Acetaminophen, 35)

Haleys M-O (See Magnesium Salts, 67)

Halfprin 81 (See Aspirin, 37)

Halls Cough Drops (See Menthol, 69)

Halotussin-DM (See Dextromethorphan, 52 and Guaifenesin, 59)

Haltran (See Ibuprofen, 60)

Hayfebrol (See Chlorpheniramine, 49 and Pseudoephedrine, 80)
HC-DermaPax (See Hydrocortisone, 59)
Head and Shoulders Dry Scalp (See Pyrithione Zinc, 82)
Head and Shoulders Intensive Treatment (See Selenium Sulfide, 85)
Head and Shoulders Shampoo (See Pyrithione Zinc, 82)
Heartline (See Aspirin, 37)
Heet (See Camphor, 45 and Capsaicin, 46)
Hematinic (See Iron, 61)
Hemorid For Women (See Pramoxine, 80)
Hem Prep (See Phenylephrine, 77 and Zinc Oxide, 90)
High Potency Pain Relievers (See Acetaminophen, 35 and
    Salicylates, 84)
High Potency Tar (See Coal Tar, 52)
Histacon (See Chlorpheniramine, 49)
Histatab Plus (See Chlorpheniramine, 49 and Phenylephrine, 77)
Histine-4,-8,-12 (See Chlorpheniramine, 49)
Histine-1, -2, -25, -50 (See Diphenhydramine, 54)
Hold (See Dextromethorphan, 52)
Hurricaine (See Benzocaine, 39)
Hydra Mag Tablets (See Aluminum Hydroxide 36, Kaolin, 62,
    and Magnesium Salts, 67)
Hydrate (See Diphenhydramine, 54)
Hydrocil Instant (See Psyllium 81)
Hydrocortisone, 59
Hydroskin (See Hydrocortisone, 59)
Hysone (See Hydrocortisone, 59)
Hytuss (See Guaifenesin, 59)

Iberet (See Iron, 61)
Ibu (See Ibuprofen, 60)
Ibufon Goo (See Ibuprofen, 60)
Ibuprofen, 60
Imodium A-D (See Loperamide, 65)

Innertabs (See Psyllium, 81and Senna, 85)
Iodex (See Povidone-Iodine, 79)
Ionil T (See Coal Tar, 52)
Ircon (See Iron, 61)
Iron, 61
Irospan (See Iron, 61)
Isodettes (See Menthol, 69)
Itch-X (See Pramoxine , 80)
Ivarest Maximum Strength (See Calamine, 43 and
    Diphenhydramine, 54)
Ivocort (See Hydrocortisone, 59)

Jiffy (See Benzocaine, 39)
Johnson's Odor-Eaters (See Tolnaftate, 87)

Kaodene Non-Narcotic (See Bismuth Subsalicylate, 40
    and Kaolin, 62)
Kaolin, 62
Kaopectate (See Attapulgite, 38)
Kao-Spen (See Kaolin, 62)
Kao-Tin (See Kaolin, 62)
Kapectin (See Kaolin, 62)
K-C (See Kaolin, 62)
Keep Alert (See Caffeine, 42)
Keep Going (See Caffeine, 42)
Ketoprofen, 63
Kid Kare (See Peudoephedrine, 80)
Kolephrin (See Acetaminophen, 35, Chlorpheniramine, 49 and
    Pseudoephedrine, 80)
Kolephrin DM (See Acetaminophen, 35, Chlorpheniramine, 49,
    Dextromethorphan, 52 and Pseudoephedrine, 80)

Kolephrin GG/DM (See Dextromethorphan, 52 and Guaifenesin, 59)
Kondremul Plain (See Mineral Oil, 71)
Konsto (See Docusate Salts, 55)
Konsyl (See Psyllium, 81)
Konsyl-D (See Psyllium, 81)
Konsyl Fiber (See Calcium Polycarbophil, 45)
Koromex (See Nonoxynol-9, 75)
K-Pek (See Attapulgite, 38)
K-Pek II (See Loperamide, 65)
Kudrox Double Strength (See Aluminum Hydroxide, 36,
    Magnesium Salts, 67 and Simethicone, 86)
Kwell (See Lindane, 64)
K-Y Plus (See Nonoxynol-9, 75)

LactAid (see Lactase, 63)
Lactase, 63
Lactrase (See Lactase, 63)
Lanabiotic (See Bacitracin, 38, Neomycin, 73, Polymixin b, 78,
    and Pramoxine, 80)
Lanacane (See Benzocaine, 39 and Resorcinol, 83)
Lanacort (See Hydrocortisone, 59)
Lavatar (See Coal Tar, 52)
L.C.D. (See Coal Tar, 52)
Legatrin PM (See Acetaminophen, and Diphenhydramine, 54)
Li Ban (See Pyrethrins with Piperonyl Butoxide, 81)
Lice-Enz (See Pyrethrins with Piperonyl Butoxide, 81)
Lidocaine, 64
Lindane, 64
Lindane Lotion and Shampoo (See Lindane, 64)
LiquiChar (See Charcoal, 52)
Liqui-Doss (See Mineral Oil, 71)
Liquiprin (See Acetaminophen, 35)
Little Bottoms (See Zinc Oxide, 90)

Malt, 68

Maltsupex (See Malt, 68)

Mapap Cold Formula (See Acetaminophen, 35, Chlorpheniramine, 49, Dextromethorphan, 52 and Pseudoephedrine, 80)

Maracid 2 (See Aluminum Hydroxide, 36 and Magnesium Salts,67)

Maranox (See Acetaminophen, 35)

Massengill Medicated Douche (See Povidone-Iodine, 79)

Meclizine, 68

Meda Cap/Tab (See Acetaminophen, 35)

Medalox Gel (See Magnesium Salts, 67)

Medicated Powdser (See Menthol, 69 and Zinc Oxide, 90)

Medicone Derma (See Benzocaine, 39 and Zinc Oxide, 90)

Medicone Ointment (See Benzocaine, 39)

Medi-Flu (See Pseudoephedrine, 80)

Mediquell (See Dextromethorphan, 52)

Medi-Quik Aerosol (See Lidocaine, 64)

Medotar (See Coal Tar, 52 and Zinc Oxide, 90)

Menadol (See Ibuprofen, 60)

Menthol, 69

Mentholatum Ointment (See Camphor, 45)

Mentholin (See Camphor, 45 and Salicylates, 84)

Merdex (See Docusate Salts, 55)

Metamucil (See Psyllium, 81)

Meted (See Salicylic Acid, 84 and Sulphur, 87)

Methyl Salicylate (See Salicylates, 84)

Methylcellulouse, 70

Mexsana Medicated (See Zinc Oxide, 90)

MG Cold Sore Formula (See Lidocaine, 64 and Menthol, 69)

MG 217 (See Coal Tar, 52)

Micatin (See Miconazole, 70)

Miconazole, 70

Micro Nefrin (See Epinephrine, 57)

Midol for Cramps (See Aspirin, 37 and Caffeine, 42)

Midol IB Cramp Relief Formula (See Ibuprofen, 60)

Midol Maximum Strength (See Ibuprofen, 60)

Midol Maximum Strength PMS (See Acetaminophen, 35,
    Pamabrom, 76, and Pyrilamine, 82)
Midol Menstrual Regular Strength Multisymptom Formula
    (See Acetaminophen, 35, Caffeine, 42 and Pyrilamine, 82)
Midol PM (See Acetaminophen, 35 and Diphenhydramine, 54)
Midol Teen (See Acetaminophen, 35 and Pamabrom, 76)
Milk of Magnesia (See Magnesium Salts, 67)
Milkinol (See Mineral Oil, 71)
Mineral Oil, 71
Min-Hema (See Iron, 61)
Minidyne (See Povidone-Iodine, 79)
Minit-Rub (See Camphor, 45, Menthol, 69 and Salicylates, 84)
Mini Two Way Action (See Ephedrine, 56 and Guaifenesin, 59)
Mobigesic (See Phenyltoloxamine, 78 and Salicylates, 84)
Mobisyl (See Salicylates, 84)
Modane (See Bisacodyl, 40)
Modane Bulk (See Psyllium, 81)
Modane Soft (See Docusate Salts, 55)
Molie (See Caffeine, 42)
Mol-Iron (See Iron, 61)
Momentum (See Aspirin, 37)
Monistat (See Miconazole, 70)
Mosco (See Salicylic Acid, 84)
Motrin IB (See Ibuprofen, 60)
Murine Plus (See Tetrahydrozoline Hydrochloride, 87)
Muro's Opcon (See Naphazoline, 71)
Mycelex (See Clotrimazole, 51)
Mycelex-3 (See Butoconazole, 41)
Myciguent (See Neomycin, 73)
Mycitracin (See Bacitracin, 38, Neomycin, 73 and Polymixin b, 78)
Mygel (See Aluminum Hydroxide, 36, Magnesium Salts, 67,
    and Simethicone, 86)
Mylanta (See Aluminum Hydroxide, 36, Magnesium Salts, 67,
    and Simethicone, 86)
Mylanta II (See Aluminum Hydroxide, 36, Magnesium Salts, 67,

Nicotine, 74

Nicotrol (See Nicotine, 74)

Nighttime Cold/Flu (See Acetaminophen, 35, Dextromethorphan, 52, Doxylamine, 56, and Pseudoephedrine, 80)

Nighttime Pamprin (See Acetaminophen, 35 and Diphenhydramine, 54)

Nil Tuss (See Chlorpheniramine, 49, Dextromethorphan, 52, and Phenylephrine, 77)

Night-Time Sleep-Aid (See Diphenhydramine, 54)

Nite Time Cold Formula (See Acetaminophen, 35, Dextromethorphan, 52, Doxylamine, 56, and Pseudoephedrine, 80)

Nizatidine, 74

No Doz (See Caffeine, 42)

Nonoxynol-9, 75

No Pain HP (see Capsaicin, 46)

Norwich (See Aspirin, 37)

Nostril (See Phenylephrine, 77)

Nostrilla (See Oxymetazoline Hydrochloride, 76)

Novahistine DMX (See Dextromethorphan, 53, Guaifenesin, 59, and Pseudoephedrine, 80)

Noxzema Clear Ups (See Salicylic Acid, 84)

Noxzema Medicated Skin Cream (See Camphor, 45 and Menthol, 69)

NP-27 (See Tolnaftate, 87)

NTZ (See Oxymetazoline Hydrochloride, 76)

Nu-Iron (See Iron, 61)

Numzit (See Benzocaine, 39 and Menthol, 69)

Nupercainal (See Dibucaine, 53)

Nupercaine (See Dibucaine, 53)

Nuprin (See Ibuprofen, 60)

Nuprin Backache (See Salicylates, 84)

Nytcold Medicine (See Acetaminophen, 35, Dextromethorphan, 52, Doxylamine, 56 and Pseudoephedrine, 80)

Nytime Cold Medicine Liquid (See Acetaminophen, 35,

Dextromethorphan, 52, Doxylamine, 56,
and Pseudoephedrine, 80)
Nytol (See Diphenhydramine, 54)

Obrical (See Calcium, 43)
Occlusal HP (See Salicylic Acid, 84)
OcuClear (See Oxymetazoline, 76)
OFF-Ezy (See Salicylic Acid, 84)
Omnicol (See Acetaminophen, 35, Caffeine, 42,
Chlorpheniramine, 49, Dextromethorphan, 52,
and Phenylephrine, 77)
Opcon-A (See Naphazoline Hydrochloride, 71)
Optigene-3 (See Tetrahydrozoline Hydrochloride, 87)
Orabase Lip (See Benzocaine, 39, Camphor, 43 and Menthol, 69)
Orabase with Benzocaine (See Benzocaine, 39)
Orajel (See Benzocaine, 39)
Orasol (See Benzocaine, 39)
Ornex No Drowsiness (See Acetaminophen, 35
and Pseudoephedrine, 80)
Ortac-DM (See Dextrmethorphan, 52, Guaifenesin, 59,
and Phenylephrine, 77)
Ortho-Gynol (See Nonoxynol-9, 75)
Orudis KT (See Ketoprofen, 63)
Os-Cal -250, -500 (See Calcium, 43)
Ostiderm (See Zinc Oxide, 90)
Overtime (See Caffeine, 42)
Oxipor VHC (See Coal Tar, 52)
Oxy Clean (See Salicylic Acid, 84)
Oxy 5 (See Benzoyl Peroxide, 39)
Oxy Medicated Cleanser (See Salicylic Acid, 84)
Oxy Wash (See Benzoyl Peroxide, 39)
Oxy-10 Maximum Strength (See Benzoyl Peroxide, 39)
Oxymetazoline Hydrochloride, 76

Oysco (See Calcium Carbonate, 44)
Oyst-Cal 500 (See Calcium, 43)

P-A-C Analgesic (See Aspirin, 37 and Caffeine, 42)
Pain and Fever (See Acetaminophen, 35)
Pain Bust-R II (See Menthol, 69 and Salicylates, 84)
Pain Doctor (See Capsaicin, 46 and Salicylates, 84)
Pain Gel Plus (See Menthol, 69)
Pain Relief (See Menthol, 69 and Salicylates, 84)
Pain Relief, Aspirin-Free (See Acetaminophen, 35)
Pain-X (See Capsaicin, 46)
Pamabrom, 76
Pamprin (See Acetaminophen, 35, Pamabrom, 76,
    and Pyrilamine, 82)
Pamprin Maximun Pain Relief (See Acetaminophen, 35,
    Pamabrom, 76 and Salicylates, 84)
Pamprin Multi-Symptom Maximum Strength
    (See Acetaminophen, 35, Pamabrom, 76, and Pyrilamine, 82)
Pan Oxyl (See Benzoyl Peroxide, 39)
Panadol (See Acetaminophen, 35)
Panex (See Acetaminophen, 35)
Panitone-500 (See Acetaminophen, 35)
Paplex Ultra (See Salicylic Acid, 84)
Para-Jel (See Benzocaine, 39)
Paratrol (See Pyrethrins with Piperonyl Butoxide, 81)
Parten (See Acetaminophen, 35)
Pazo (See Ephedrine, 56 and Zinc Oxide, 90)
Pecto-Kalin (See Kaolin, 62)
PediaCare Cough-Cold (See Chlorpheniramine, 49,
    Dextromethorphan, 52, and Pseudoephedrine, 80)
PediaCare Cough-Cold Formula (See Dextromethorphan, 52
    and Pseudoephedrine, 80)
PediaCare Night Rest Cough-Cold Formula

(See Chlorpheniramine, 49, Dextromethorphan, 52,
and Pseudoephedrine, 80)

Pentrax (See Coal Tar, 52)

Pentrax Gold (See Coal Tar, 52)

Pep-Back (See Caffeine, 42)

Pepcid (See Famotidine, 57)

Pepcid Complete (See Calcium Carbonate, 44, Famotidine, 57,
and Magnesium Salts, 67)

Peptic Relief (See Bismuth Subsalicylate, 40)

Pepto-Bismol (See Bismuth Subsalicylate, 40)

Percogesic (See Acetaminophen, 35 and Phenyltoloxamine, 78)

Percogesic Extra Strength (See Acetaminophen, 35
and Diphenhydramine, 54)

Percy Medicine (See Bismuth Subsalicylate, 40)

Perdiem (See Psyllium, 81 and Senna, 85)

Peri-Colace (See Casanthranol, 46 and Docusate Salts, 55)

Peri-Dos (See Casanthranol, 46 and Docusate Salts, 55)

Pernox (See Salicylic Acid, 84 and Sulphur, 87)

Peroxin (See Benzoyl Peroxide, 39)

Pertussin (See Dextromethorphan, 52)

Pertussin All Night PM (See Acetaminophen, 35,
Dextromethorphan, 52, Doxylamine, 56 and
Pseudoephedrine, 80)

Pertussin CS (See Dextromethorphan, 52 and Guaifenesin, 59)

Pertussin ES (See Dextromethorphan, 52)

Phanatuss (See Dextromethorphan, 52 and Guaifenesin, 59)

Phazyme (See Simethicone, 86)

Phenazopyridine Hydrochloride, 77

Phenylephrine, 77

Phenylgesic (See Acetaminophen, 35 and Phenyltoloxamine, 78)

Phillips' Chewable (See Magnesium Salts, 67)

Phillips' LaxCaps (See Docusate Salts, 55)

Phillips' Liquigels (See Docusate Salts, 55)

Phillips' Milk of Magnesia (See Magnesium Salts, 67)

Pinex Cough (See Dextromethorphan, 52)

Plexolan Lanolin (See Zinc Oxide, 90)
Poldeman (See Kaolin, 62)
Poldemicina (See Kaolin, 62)
Polydine (See Povidone-Iodine, 79)
Polymyxin b, 78
Polysporin (See Bacitracin, 38 and Polymyxin b, 78)
Polytar (See Coal Tar, 52)
Poslam Psoriasis (See Salicylic Acid, 84 and Sulphur, 87)
Posture (See Calcium, 43)
Povidone-Iodine, 79
PrameGel (See Menthol, 69 and Pramoxine Hydrochloride, 80)
Pramoxine Hydrochloride, 80
Prax (See Pramoxine Hydrochloride, 80)
Premsyn (See Acetaminophen, 35 and Pyrilamine, 82)
Preparation-H (See Phenylephrine, 77)
Presalin (See Acetaminophen, 35, Aluminum Hydroxide, 36,
    and Aspirin, 37)
Primatene (See Ephedrine, 56 and Guaifenesin, 59)
Primatene Mist (See Epinephrine, 57)
Primatuss Cough Mixture 4D (See Dextromethorphan, 52,
    Guaifenesin, 59 and Pseudoephedrine, 80)
Privine (See Naphazoline Hydrochloride, 71)
Procort (See Hydrocortisone, 59)
Procto Foam HC (See Hydrocortisone, 59 and Pramoxine
    Hydrochloride, 80)
Pronemia Hematinic (See Iron, 61)
Pronto-Lice Killing Shampoo (See Pyrethrins with Piperonyl
    Butoxide, 81)
Propa pH (See Salicylic Acid, 84)
Pro-Sof (See Casanthranol, 46)
Pro-Sof Plus (See Casanthranol, 46 and Docusate Salts, 55)
Prostep (See Nicotine, 74)
Pseudoephedrine, 80
Pseudo-Phedrine (See Pseudoephedrine, 80)
Pseudo Plus (See Chlorpheniramine, 49 and Pseudoephedrine, 80)

Pseudo Syrup (See Pseudoephedrine, 80)
Psorigel (See Coal Tar, 52)
PsoriNail (See Coal Tar, 52)
Psyllium, 81
Purge (See Castol Oil, 48)
Pyrethrins with Piperonyl Butoxide, 81
Pyrinex (See Pyrethrins with Piperonyl Butoxide, 81)
Pyrithione Zinc, 82

Quiecof (See Chlorpheniramine, 49 and Dextromethorphan, 52)
Quiet World (See Acetaminophen, 35 and Pyrilamine, 81)
Quik-Pep (See Caffeine, 42)

Ranitidine, 83
Rectal Medicone (See Benzocaine, 39)
Refenesen Plus (See Guaifenesin, 59 and Pseudoephedrine, 80)
Regulax SS (See Docusate Salts, 55)
Reguloid (See Psyllium, 81)
Reliable Gentle Laxative (See Bisacodyl, 40)
REM (See Dextromethorphan, 52)
Renpap (See Acetaminophen, 35, Caffeine, 42 and Salicylates, 84)
Rescon-DM (See Chlorpheniramine, 49, Dextromethorphan, 52,
    and Phenylephrine, 77)
Rescon-GG (See Chlorpheniramine, 49 and Pseudoephedrine, 80)
Resinol (See Calamine, 43 and Zinc Oxide, 90)
Resorcinol, 83
Rest Easy (See Acetaminophen, 35, Dextromethorphan, 52,
    Doxylamine, 56 and Pseudoephedrine, 80)
Rezamid (See Resorcinol, 83 and Sulphur, 87)
R-Gel (See Capsaicin, 46)
Rheaban (See Attapulgite, 38)

Rhinall (See Phenylephrine, 77)

Rhinosyn-DM (See Chlorpheniramine, 49, Dextromethorphan, 52, and Pseudoephedrine, 80)

Rhinosyn-X (See Dextromethorphan, 52, Guaifenesin, 59, and Pseudoephedrine, 80)

Rhuli Gel (See Camphor, 45 and Menthol, 69)

Rhuli Spray (See Benzocaine, 39, Calamine, 43, Camphor, 45, and Menthol, 69)

RID (See Pyrethrins with Piperonyl Butoxide, 81)

Rid-a-Pain Cream (See Capsaicin, 46)

Riopan (See Magaldrate, 66)

Riopan Plus (See Magaldrate, 66 and Simethicone, 86)

Robafen (See Guaifenesin, 59)

Robafen CF (See Dextromethorphan, 52, Guaifenesin, 59, and Pseudoephedrine, 80)

Robafen DM (See Dextromethorphan, 52 and Guaifenesin, 59)

Robitussin (See Guaifenesin, 59)

Robitussin Allergy & Cough (See Brompheniramine, 41, Dextromethorphan, 52 and Pseudoephedrine, 80)

Robitussin-CF (See Dextromethorphan, 52, Guaifenesin, 59, and Pseudoephedrine, 80)

Robitussin Cold Cold & Congestion (See Dextromethorphan, 52, Guaifenesin, 59 and Pseudoephedrine, 80)

Robitussin Cold Multi-Symptom Cold & Flu (See Acetaminophen, 35, Dextromethorphan, 52, Guaifenesin, 59, and Pseudoephedrine, 80)

Robitussin Cold Severe Congestion (See Guaifenesin, 59 and Pseudoephedrine, 80)

Robitussin Cough Drops (See Dextromethorphan, 52)

Robitussin DM (See Guaifenesin, 59 and Dextromethorphan, 52)

Robitussin Flu (See Acetaminophen, 35, Chlorpheniramine, 49, Dextromethorphan, 52 and Pseudoephedrine, 80)

Robitussin Honey Calmers Throat Drops (See Menthol, 69)

Robitussin Honey Cough (See Dextromethorphan, 52)

Robitussin Honey Cough Drops (See Menthol, 69)

Robitussin Honey Flu Nighttime Formula (See Acetaminophen, 35, Chlorpheniramine, 49, Dextromethorphan, 52, and Pseudoephedrine, 80)

Robitussin Maximum Strength Cough & Cold (See Dextromethorphan, 52 and Pseudoephedrine, 80)

Robitussin Maximum Strength Cough Suppressant (See Dextromethorphan, 52)

Robitussin Multi-Symptom Honey Flu (See Acetaminophen, 35, Dextromethorphan, 52 and Pseudoephedrine, 80)

Robitussin PE (See Guaifenesin, 59 and Pseudoephedrine, 80)

Robitussin Sinus & Congestion (See Acetaminophen, 35, Guaifenesin, 59, and Pseudoephedrine, 80)

Robitussin Sugar-Free Cough (See Dextromethorphan, 52 and Guaifenesin, 59)

Rolaids Calcium Rich (See Calcium Carbonate, 44 and Magnesium Salts, 67)

Romach Antacid (See Magnesium Salts, 67 and Sodium Bicarbonate, 86)

Rulox (See Aluminum Hydroxide, 36 and Magnesium Salts, 67)

Rymed (See Guaifenesin, 59 and Pseudoephedrine, 80)

Ryna (See Chlorpheniramine, 49 and Pseudoephedrine, 80)

Safe Tussin (See Dextromethorphan, 52 and Guaiafenesin, 59)

SalAc Cleanser (See Salicylic Acid, 84)

Sal-Acid Wart Remover (See Salicylic Acid, 84)

Salactic Film (See Salicylic Acid, 84)

Saleto (See Acetaminophen, Aspirin, 37 and Caffeine, 42)

Saleto 200 (See Ibuprofen, 60)

Salicylates, 84

Salicylic Acid, 84

Salicylic Acid and Sulfur Soap (See Sulphur, 87 and Salicylic Acid, 84)

Sal-Plant (See Salicylic Acid, 84)

Sarna (See Camphor, 45 and Menthol, 69)

SAStid (See Sulphur, 87)

Scalpicin (See Menthol, 69 and Salicylic Acid, 84)

Schamberg's Anti-Itch (See Menthol, 69 and Zinc Oxide, 90)

Scotcof (See Chlorpheniramine, 49, Dextromethorphan, 52, Guaifenesin, 59 and Phenylephrine, 77)

Scot-Tussin Allergy Relief Formula (See Diphenhydramine, 54 and Menthol, 69)

Scot-Tussin DM (See Chlorpheniramine, 49 and Dextromethorphan, 52)

Scot-Tussin Expectorant (See Guaifenesin, 59 and Menthol, 69)

Scot-Tussin Hayfebrol (See Chlorpheniramine, 49, Menthol, 69, and Pseudoephedrine, 80)

Scot-Tussin Pharmacal Allergy (See Diphenhydramine, 54)

Scot-Tussin Pharmacal DM (See Chlorpheniramine, 49 and Dextromethorphan, 52)

Scot-Tussin Senior Clear (See Dextromethorphan, 52 and Guaifenesin, 59)

Sebasorb (See Attapulgite, 38 and Salicylic Acid, 84)

Sebex-T (See Coal Tar, 52 and Sulphur, 87)

Sebulex (See Sulphur, 87)

Sebulon (See Pyrithione Zinc, 82)

Sebutone (See Coal Tar, 52 and Sulphur, 87)

Selenium Sulfide, 85

Selsun Blue (See Selenium Sulfide, 85)

Semicid Inserts (See Nonoxynol-9, 75)

Senexon (See Senna, 85)

Senna, 85

Senna-Gen (See Senna, 85)

Senokot (See Senna, 85)

Senokot S (See Docusate Salts, 55 and Senna, 85)

SensoGARD (See Benzocaine, 39)

Serutan (See Psyllium, 81)

Shur-Seal (See Nonoxynol-9, 75)

Signate (See Dimenhydrinate, 53)

Silace (See Docusate Salts, 55)

Silace-C (See Casanthranol, 46)
Silafed (See Pseudoephedrine, 80 and Triprolidine, 88)
Siladryl (See Diphenhydramine, 54)
Silphen Cough (See Diphenhydramine, 54)
Silphen DM (See Dextromethorphan, 52)
Siltussin (See Guaifenesin, 59)
Simethicone, 86
Simplet (See Acetaminophen, 35, Chlorpheniramine, 49,
    and Pseudoephedrine, 80)
Simply Sleep (See Diphenhydramine, 54)
Sinarest Decongestant (See Oxymetazoline Hydrochloride, 76)
Sinarest Extra-Strength (See Acetaminophen, 35,
    Chlorpheniramine, 49 and Pseudoephedrine, 80)
Sinarest Sinus (See Acetaminophen, 35, Chlorpheniramine, 49,
    and Pseudoephedrine, 80)
Sine-Aid IB (See Ibuprofen, 60 and Pseudoephedrine, 80)
Sine-Aid Maximum Strength (See Acetaminophen, 35
    and Pseudoephedrine, 80)
Sine-Off No Drowsiness (See Acetaminophen, 35
    and Pseudoephedrine, 80)
Sine-Off Sinus Medicine (See Acetaminophen, 35,
    Chlorpheniramine, 49 and Pseudoephedrine, 80)
Sinex (See Phenylephrine, 77)
Singlet (See Acetaminophen, 35, Chlorpheniramine, 49,
    and Pseudoephedrine, 80)
Sinus Headache & Congestion (See Acetaminophen, 35,
    Chlorpheniramine, 49, and Pseudoephedrine, 80)
Sinus Relief (See Acetaminophen, 35 and Pseudoephedrine, 80)
Sinus Tablets (See Acetaminophen, 35, Chlorpheniramine, 49,
    and Pseudoephedrine, 80)
Sinustop (See Pseudoephedrine, 80)
Sinutab Non-Drying (See Guaifenesin, 59 and Pseudoephdrine, 80)
Sinutab Sinus Allergy Medication Maximum Strength
    (See Acetaminophen, 35, Chlorpheniramine, 49,
    and Pseudoephedrine, 80)

Sleep Cap (See Diphenhydramine, 54)
Sleep-Eze 3 (See Diphenhydramine, 54)
Sleep II (See Diphenhydramine, 54)
Sloan's (See Capsaicin, 46 and Salicylates, 84)
Slo-Fe (See Iron, 61)
SLT Lotion (See Coal Tar, 52 and Salicylic Acid, 84)
Snaplets-D (See Chlorpheniramine, 49 and Pseudoephedrine, 80)
Snaplets-FR (See Acetaminophen, 35)
Snooze Fast (See Diphenhydramine, 54)
Sodium Bicarbonate, 86
Sodium Salicylate (See Salicylates, 84)
Soft'n Soothe (See Benzocaine, 39 and Menthol, 69)
Solarcaine (See Benzocaine, 39)
Solarcaine Aloe Extra Burn Relief (See Lidocaine, 64)
Soltice Quick Rub (See Camphor, 45, Menthol, 69 and Salicylates, 84)
Sominex (See Diphenhydramine, 54)
Soothe (See Tetrahydrozoline Hydrochloride, 87)
Sorbase Cough (See Dextromethorphan, 52 and Guaifenesin, 59)
Spectro-Biotic (See Bacitracin, 38, Neomycin, 73 and Polymixin b, 78)
Spectrocin Plus (See Bacitracin, 38, Neomycin, 73 Pramoxine, 80,
    and Polymixin b, 78)
Spec-T Sore Throat Anesthetic (See Benzocaine, 39)
Spec-T Sore Throat Cough Suppressant (See Benzocaine, 39
    and Dextromethorphan, 52)
Sports Spray Extra Strength (See Camphor, 45, Menthol, 69,
    and Salicylates, 84)
Sportscreme (See Salicylates, 84)
Stay Alert (See Caffeine, 42)
Stay Awake (See Caffeine, 42)
StePhan Relief Capsules (See Psyllium, 81)
St. Joseph Aspirin (See Aspirin, 37)
St. Joseph Cough Suppressant (See Dextromethorphan, 52)
Stool Softener DC (See Docusate Salts, 55)
Stri-Dex B.P. (See Benzoyl Peroxide, 39)
Stri-Dex Clear (See Salicylic Acid, 84)

Stri-Dex Lotion (See Salicylic Acid, 84)
Stuart Hematinic (See Iron, 61)
Stulex (See Docusate Salts, 55)
Sucrets 4-Hour Cough (See Dextromethorphan, 52 and Menthol, 69)
Sudafed Decongestant (4, 12 & 24 hour) Tablets
    (See Pseudoephedrine, 80)
Sudafed Cold and Cough (See Actaminophen, 35,
    Dextromethorphan, 52, Guaifenesin, 59,
    and Pseudoephedrine, 80)
Sudafed Non-Drying Non-Drowsy MS Liquid Caps
    (See Guaifenesin, 59 and Pseudoephedrine, 80)
Sudafed Severe Cold Caplets (See Acetaminophen, 35,
    Dextromethorphan, 52 and Pseudoephedrine, 80)
Sudafed Sinus & Allergy (See Chlorpheniramine, 49
    and Pseudoephedrine, 80)
Sudafed Sinus & Cold (See Actaminophen, 35
    and Pseudoephedrine, 80)
Sudafed Sinus Headache (See Actaminophen, 35
    and Pseudoephedrine, 80)
Sudafed Sinus Nighttime (See Pseudoephedrine, 80
    and Triprolidine, 88)
SudoGest Sinus (See Acetaminophen, 35 and
    Pseodoephedrine, 80)
Sudrin (See Pseudoephedrine, 80)
Sulfoam Medicated Antidandruff (See Sulphur, 87)
Sulforcin (See Resorcinol, 83 and Sulphur, 87)
Sulmasque (See Sulphur, 87)
Sulpho-Lac (See Sulphur, 87)
Sulphur, 87
Sulray Acne (See Sulphur, 87)
Sulray Aloe Vera Skin Protectant (See Zinc Oxide, 90)
Summer's Eve Medicated Douche (See Povidone-Iodine, 79)
Summit Extra Strength (See Acetaminophen, 35, Aspirin, 37,
    and Caffeine, 42)
Suppap-120, -325, -650, (See Acetaminophen, 35)

SureLac (See Lactase, 63)
Surfak (See Docusate Salts, 55)
Surpass (See Calcium Carbonate, 44)
Swiss Kriss (See Senna, 85)
Syllact (See Psyllium, 81)
Synacol CF (See Dextromethorphan, 52 and Guaifenesin, 59)
Synatuss-One (See Dextromethorphan, 52 and Guaifenesin, 59)

Tagamet HB (See Cimetidine, 49)
Tanac (See Benzocaine, 39)
Tar Paste (See Coal Tar, 52)
Tarsum Shampoo/Gel (See Coal Tar, 52 and Salicylic Acid, 84)
Tavist Allergy (See Clemastine, 50)
Tavist Sinus (See Acetaminophen, 35 and Pseudoephedrine, 80)
Tegrin Medicated Shampoo (See Coal Tar, 52)
Teldrin (See Chlorpheniramine, 49)
Temetan (See Acetaminophen, 35)
Tempo (See Aluminum Hydroxide, 36, Calcium Carbonate, 44,
    Magnesium Salts, 67 and Simethicone, 86)
Tempra (See Acetaminophen, 35)
Tetrahydrozoline Hydrochloride, 87
Therac (See Sulphur, 87)
TheraFlu Cold and Cough Nighttime (See Acetaminophen, 35,
    Chlorpheniramine, 49, Dextromethorphan, 52,
    and Pseudoephedrine, 80)
TheraFlu Cold & Sore Throat Nighttime (See Acetaminophen, 35,
    Chlorpheniramine, 49 and Pseudoephedrine, 80)
TheraFlu Maximum Strength Flu and Congestion
    (See Acetaminophen, 35, Guaifenesin, 59, Dextromethorphan,
    52, and Pseudoephedrine, 80)
TheraFlu Maximum Strength Flu & Cough Nighttime
    (See Acetaminophen, 35, Chlorpheniramine, 49,
    Dextromethorphan, 52 and Pseudoephedrine, 80)

TheraFlu Maximum Strength Flu & Sore Throat Nighttime
(See Acetaminophen, 35, Chlorpheniramine, 49,
and Pseudoephedrine, 80)
TheraFlu Maximum Strength Severe Cold & Congestion Nighttime
(See Acetaminophen, 35, Chlorpheniramine, 49,
Dextromethorphan, 52 and Pseudoephedrine, 80)
TheraFlu Maximum Strength Severe Cold & Congestion
Non-Drowsy (See Acetaminophen, 35, Dextromethorphan, 52,
and Pseudoephedrine, 80)
Thera-Gesic Crème (See Menthol, 69 and Salicylates, 84)
TheraPatch Cold Sore (See Camphor, 45 and Lidocaine, 64)
Thylox (See Sulphur, 87)
Tigo (See Bacitracin, 38, Neomycin, 73 and Polymixin b, 78)
Tinactin (See Tolnaftate, 87)
Ting Antifungal (See Miconazole, 70)
Tisit (See Pyrethrins with Piperonyl Butoxide, 81)
Titralac (See Calcium Carbonate, 44)
Titralac Plus (See Calcium Carbonate, 44 and Simethicone, 86)
Tolnaftate, 87
Tolu-Sed DM (See Dextromethorphan, 52 and Guaifenesin, 59)
Toothache (See Benzocaine, 39)
Top Care LiquiCaps Nite Time Multi-Symtom Cold/Flu Relief
(See Acetaminophen, 35, Dextromethorphan, 52, Doxylamine,
56, and Pseudoephedrine, 80)
Top Care Maximum Strength Flu Cold & Cough Medicine Night
Time (See Acetaminophen, 35, Chlorpheniramine, 49,
Dextromethorphan, 52 and Pseudoephedrine, 80)
Top Care Maximum Strength Soothing Cough & Head Congestion
Relief D (See Dextromethorphan, 52 and Pseudoephedrine, 80)
Top Care Multi-Symptom Pain Relief Cold (See Acetaminophen,
35, Dextromethorphan, 52 and Pseudoephedrine, 80)
Tranquils Tablets (See Acetaminophen, 35 and Pyrilamine, 82)
Trans-Ver-Sal (See Salicylic Acid, 84)
Traveltabs (See Dimenhydrinate, 53)
Triacting Cold & Allergy (See Chlorpheniramine, 49

and Pseudoephedrine, 80)

Triaminic Allergy Congestion (See Pseudoephedrine, 80)

Triaminic Allergy Sinus & Headache (See Chlorpheniramine, 49)

Triaminic Cold & Allergy (See Chlorpheniramine, 49 and
    Pseudoephedrine, 80)

Triaminic Cold & Cough (See Chlorpheniramine, 49,
    Dextromethorphan, 52, and Pseudoephedrine , 80)

Triaminic Cold & Nighttime Cough (See Chlorpheniramine, 49,
    Dextromethorphan, 52 and Pseudoephedrine, 80)

Triaminic Cough Liquid (See Dextromethorphan, 52 and
    Pseudoephedrine, 80)

Triaminic Cough & Congestion Liquid (See Dextromethorphan,
    52 and Pseudoephedrine, 80)

Triaminic Flu Cough & Fever (See Acetaminophen, 35,
    Chlorpheniramine, 49, Dextromethorphan, 52 and
    Pseudoephedrine, 80)

Tri-Biozene (See Bacitracin, 38, Neomycin, 73, Polymixin b, 78,
    and Pramoxine, 80)

Tricodene Liquid (See Dextromethorphan, 52 and
    Chlorpheniramine, 49)

Tricodene Sugar Free (See Chlorpheniramine, 49,
    Dextromethorphan, 52 and Menthol, 69)

Trimixin (See Bacitracin, 38, Neomycin, 73 and Polymixin b, 78)

Triple Antibiotic (See Bacitracin, 38, Neomycin, 73,
    and Polymixin b, 78)

Triple X (See Pyrethrins with Piperonyl Butoxide, 81)

Triprolidine, 88

Triptone (See Dimenhydrinate, 53)

Trocaine (See Benzocaine, 39)

Trolamine Salicylate, 84

Tronolane Cream (See Pramoxine Hydrochloride, 80)

Tronolane Suppositories (See Zinc Oxide, 90)

Tronothane Hydrochloride (See Pramoxine Hydrochloride, 80)

T/Scalp (See Hydrocortisone, 59)

Tums (See Calcium Carbonate, 44)

Tums Plus (See Calcium Carbonate, 44 and Simethicone, 86)

Tusibron (See Guaifenesin, 59)

Tussex Cough (See Dextromethorphan, 52, Guaifenesin, 59, and Phenylephrine, 77)

Twice-A-Day 12-Hour Nasal Spray (See Oxymetazoline, 76)

Twilite (See Diphenhydramine, 54)

Ty-Caps (See Acetaminophen, 35)

Ty-Cold Formula (See Acetaminophen, 35, Chlorpheniramine, 49, Dextromethorphan, 52 and Pseudoephedrine, 80)

Tylenol (See Actaminophen, 35)

Tylenol Allergy Sinus (See Acetaminophen, 35, Chlorpheniramine, 49, and Pseudoephedrine, 80)

Tylenol Allergy Sinus Maximum Strength (See Acetaminophen, 35, Chlorpheniramine, 49 and Pseudoephedrine, 80)

Tylenol Allergy Sinus Nighttime Maximum-Strength (See Acetaminophen, 35, Diphenhydramine, 54, and Pseudoephedrine, 80)

Tylenol Arthritis Pain Extended Relief (See Acetaminophen, 35)

Tylenol Cold Multi-Symptom Complete Formula (See Acetaminophen, 35, Chlorpheniramine, 49, Dextromethorphan, 52 and Pseudoephedrine, 80)

Tylenol Cold Multi-Symptom Non-Drowsy (See Acetaminophen, 35, Dextromethorphan, 52 and Pseudoephedrine, 80)

Tylenol Cold Multi-Symptom Severe Congestion (See Acetaminophen, 35, Dextromethorphan, 52, Guaifenesin, 59, and Pseudoephedrine, 80)

Tylenol Flu Maximum Strength Nighttime (See Acetaminophen, 35, Diphenhydramine, 54 and Pseudeoephedrine, 80)

Tylenol Flu Maximum Strength Non-Drowsy (See Acetamiophen, 35, Dextromethorphan, 52, and Pseudoephedrine, 80)

Tylenol PM Extra Strength (See Acetaminophen, 35 and Diphenhydramine, 54)

Tylenol Severe Allergy (See Acetaminophen, 35 and Diphenhydramine, 54)

Tylenol Sinus Maximum Strength Nighttime (See Acetaminophen,

35, Doxylamine, 56 and Pseudoephedrine, 80)
Tylenol Sinus Maximum Strength Non-Drowsy
(See Acetaminophen, 35 and Pseudoephedrine, 80)
Tylenol Sore Throat Maximum Strength (See Acetaminophen, 35)
Tylenol Women's Menstrual Relief (See Acetaminophen, 35)
Ty-Pap (See Acetaminophen, 35)
Ty-Tabs (See Acetaminophen, 35)

Undecylenate Salts, 88
Undelenic Ointment (See Undecylenate Salts, 88)
Unisom Night-Time Sleep Aid (See Doxylamine, 56)
Unisom With Pain Relief (See Acetaminophen, 35 and
Diphenhydramine, 54)
Uromag (See Magnesium Salts, 67)

Vagisil (See Benzocaine, 39 and Resorcinol, 83)
Valentine (See Caffeine, 42)
Vanoxide (See Benzoyl Peroxide, 39)
Vanquish (See Acetaminophen, 35, Aluminum Hydroxide 36,
Aspirin, 37, Caffeine, 42 and Magnesium Salts, 67)
Vanseb T (See Coal Tar, 52)
Vaso Clear (See Naphazoline Hydrochloride, 71)
Vasocon-A (See Naphazoline Hydrochloride, 71)
VCF (See Nonoxynol-9, 75)
Vergon (See Meclizine, 68)
Vertab (See Dimenhydrinate, 53)
Vicks 44 Cough Relief (See Dextromethorphan, 52)
Vicks 44D Cough and Head Congestion Relief
(See Dextromethorphan, 52 and Pseudoephedrine, 80)
Vicks 44E Cough and Chest Congestion Relief
(See Dextromethorphan, 52 and Guaifenesin, 59)

137

Vicks 44M Cough, Cold and Flu Relief (See Acetaminophen, 35,
   Chlorpheniramine, 49, Dextromethorphan, 52 and
   Pseudoephedrine, 80)
Vicks Cough Drops (See Menthol, 69)
Vicks DayQuil LiquiCaps Multi-Symptom Cold/Flu Relief
   (See Acetaminophen, 35, Dextromethorphan, 52 and
   Pseudoephedrine, 80)
Vicks NyQuil Cough Liquid (See Dextromethorphan, 52 and
   Doxylamine, 56)
Vicks NyQuil Liquicaps Multi-Symptom Cold/Flu Relief
   (See Acetaminophen, 35, Dextromethorphan, 52, Doxylamine,
   56 and Pseudoephedrine, 80)
Vicks Sinex Nasal Spray (See Phenylephrine, 77)
Vicks Sinex 12-Hour Nasal Spray (See Oxymetazoline, 76)
Vicks VapoRub (See Camphor, 45 and Menthol, 69)
Vicks VapoSteam (See Camphor, 45)
Victor's (See Menthol, 69)
Viro-Med (See Acetaminophen, 35, Chlorpheniramine, 49,
   Dextromethorphan, 52 and Pseudoephedrine, 80)
Visine A Eye Drops (See Naphazoline, 71)
VitaHist Oral Spray (See Dimenhydrinate, 53)
Vitamins, 89
Vitelle Lurline PMS (See Acetaminophen, 35 and Pamabrom, 76)
Vivarin (See Caffeine, 42)

Wal-Tussin (See Guaifenesin, 59)
Wart-Off (See Salicylic Acid, 84)
Woman's Gentle Laxative (See Bisacodyl, 40)
Wyanoids (See Zinc Oxide, 90)

X-Prep (See Senna, 85)

Zantac (See Ranitidine, 83)
Zeasorb-AF (See Miconazole, 70)
Zetar (See Coal Tar, 52)
Zilactin-B (See Benzocaine, 39)
Zilactin-L (See Lidocaine, 64)
Zinc Oxide, 90
Zincon (See Pyrithione Zinc, 82)
ZNP Bar (See Pyrithione Zinc, 82)

20/20 (See Caffeine, 42)
357 Magnum II (See Caffeine, 42)

References

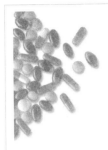

American College of Obstetrics and Gynecology, Planning Your Pregnancy and Birth, 3rd Edition, 2000.

American Drug Index, 2003: 47th Edition, Billups, N.F. and Billups, S.M., editors, Facts And Comparison, 2002.

Brent RL: Teratogen update: Bendectin. Teratology 31:429, 1985. Editorial.

Brent RL: The Bendectin saga: Another American Tragedy. Teratology 27:283, 1983. Editorial.

Briggs GG, Freeman RK, Yaffe SJ, Drugs in Pregnancy and Lactation, 6th ed., Baltimore, Williams and Wilkins, 2002.

Burrow GN: Thyroid Diseases. p. 229. In Burrow GN Ferris TF (eds): Medical Complications During Pregnancy. WB Saunders, Philadelphia, 1988.

Cunningham FG, Gant NF, Leveno KJ, Gilstrap LC, Hauth JC, Wenstrom KD, eds., Williams Obstetrics, 21st Ed., Norwalk, Conn., Appleton and Lange, 2001.

Food and Drug Administration Drug Bulletin: Pregnancy Categories for Prescription Drugs. September 1979.

Gabbe S.G., Niebyl JR, Simpson JL, eds., Obstetrics: Normal and Problem Pregnancies, 2nd Ed., New York Churchill Livingstone; 1991.

Gleicher N, Ed., Medical Therapy in Pregnancy, 2nd Ed., Norwalk, Conn, Appleton and Lange, 1992.

Griffith W.H. M.D., The Complete Guide to Vitamins, Minerals, and Supplements; Tucson, AZ: Fisher Books; 1988.

Hale T, Medications and Mothers' Milk, 10th Edition, Pharmasoft Publishing, 2002.

Heinonen OP, Slone D, Shapiro S: Birth Defects and Drugs in Pregnancy, Littleton, MA, John Wright-Publishing Sciences Group, 1983.

Hickok DE, Hollenbach KA, Reilley SF, Nyberg DA: The Association Between Decreased Amniotic Fluid Volume and Treatment with Nonsteroidal Anti-Inflammatory Agents for Preterm Labor. Am J Obstet Gynecol 160:1525, 1989.

Kowalchik C., Hylton WH., eds., Rodale's Illustrated Encyclopedia of Herbs. Emmaus, PA: Rodale Press; 1987.

Lust J., The Herb Book. New York: Bantam Books; 1974.

Mills JL, Graubard BI: Is Moderate Drinking During Pregnancy Associated with an Increased Risk of Malformations? Pediatrics 80:309, 1987.

Mills JL, Reed GF, Nugent RP et al: Are There Adverse Effects of Periconceptional Spermicide Use? Fertil Steril 43:442, 1985.

Olin BR. ed., The Lawrence Review of Natural Products. St. Louis, MO: J.B. Lippincolt Company; 1990.

PDR for Herbal Medicines, Montvale, NJ, Medical Economics Co., 2000.

Physicians' Desk Reference, 57th ed., Montvale, NJ, Medical Economics Co., 2003.

Physicians' Desk Reference for Nonprescription Drugs and Dietary Supplements, 23rd ed, Montvale NJ, Thompson Medical Economics, 2002.

Rapp RP, ed., The Pill Book Guide to Over-the-Counter Medications, New York, Bantam Books, 1997.

Rosa FW, Baum C, Shaw M: Pregnancy Outcomes After First Trimester Vaginitis Drug Therapy. Obstet Gynecol 69:751, 1987.

Rosenfeld I, Dr. Rosenfeld's Guide to Alternative Medicine. New York, Random House, 1996.

Scialli AR, Lione A, Padgett GKB, Reproductive Effects of Chemical, Physical and Biologic Agents, Reprotox, Baltimore, Johns Hopkins University Press, 1995.

Shapiro S, Slone D, Heinonen OP et al: Birth Defects and Vaginal Spermicides. JAMA 247:2381, 1982.

The USP Guide to Medicines, 1st ed., New York, Avon Books, 1996.

Wallenburg HCS, Dekker GA, Makovitz JW et al: Low-Dose Aspirin Prevents Pregnancy-Induced Hypertension and Preeclampsia in Angiotensin-Sensitive Primigravidae. Lancet 1:1, 1986.

Wilson JG, Fraser FC (eds): Handbook of Teratology. Plenum Press, New York, 1979.

Brand Names*

*Not all brands are listed

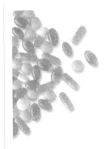

GENERIC MEDICATION: Acetaminophen

BRAND NAMES:

Aceta, Actamin, Aminofen, Apap, Arthritis Foundation Aspirin Free, Aspirin Free Pain Relief, Bayer Select Aspirin-Free, Dapa, Dolono, Dorcol, Extra Strength Dynafed E.X, Feverall, Genapap, Genebs, Halenol, Liquiprin, Meda Cap, Meda Tab, Neopap, Panadol, Panex, Panitone-500, Parten, Suppap-120, 325, 650, Temetan, Tempra, Ty-caps, Ty-Pap, Ty-Tabs, Tylenol medications

ACETAMINOPHEN IN COMBINATIONS:

Acid-X, Actifed Cold & Sinus Maximum Strength, Actifed Plus, Actifed Sinus Daytime/Nighttime, Alka-Seltzer Plus Cold, Allerest No Drowsiness, Allerest Sinus Pain Formula, Bayer Select Aspirin-Free, Benadryl Allergy & Cold, Benadryl Allergy & Sinus Headache, Benadryl Maximum Strength Severe Allergy & Sinus Headache, Bromo Seltzer, Cepacol Sore Throat, CoApap, Codimal, Coldrine, Comtrex Medications, Contac medications, Coricidin HBP Cold & Flu, Coricidin Plus, CoTylenol Cold Formula, Dimetapp Non-Drowsy Flu, Dristan Cold, Drixoral Cold & Flu, Dryphen Multi-Symptom, Excedrin Aspirin Free, Excedrin Extra Strength, Excedrine Sinus, FemBack, Fem-1, Fendol, Flextra-DS, Genacol Maximum Strength Cold & Flu Relief, Gendecon, Genite, Good Sense, Goody's, Kolephrin, Kolephrin/DM, Legatrin PM, Liquiprin, Major-gesic, Mapap, Maximum Strength Dynafed Plus,

Midol Maximum Strength, Midol Maximum Strength Menstrual, Midol PM, Midol Teen, Multi-Symptom Tylenol Cough, Multi-Symptom Tylenol Cough with Congestant, Naldegesic, N-D Gesic, Nite Time Cold Formula, Ornex, Pamprin, Phenylgesic, Quiet World, Robitussin Cold Multi-Symptom Cold & Flu, Saleto, Saleto D, Simplet, Sinarest, Sine-Aid Maximum Strength, Sine-Off medications, Singlet for Adults, Sinus-Relief, Sinutab, Sinutab Sinus Allergy Maximum Strength, Sinutab Sinus Without Drowsiness, Sudafed Cold & Cough, SudoGest Sinus, Summit Extra Strength, Tavist Allergy/Sinus/Headache, Tavist Sinus Maximum Strength, TheraFlu medications, Top Care medications, Triaminic Flu, Cough & Fever, Vanquish, Vicks DayQuil, Vicks 44M Cough Cold & Flu Relief, Vicks NyQuil Multi-Symptom Cold & Flu Relief, Viro-Med, Vitelle Lurline PMS

GENERIC MEDICATION: Aluminum Hydroxide

BRAND NAMES:

AlternaGel, Alu-Cap, Al-U-Crème, Alu-tab, Amphojel, Maalox HRF

ALUMINUM HYDROXIDE IN COMBINATIONS:

Aludrox, Alurex, Arcodex, Ascriptin, Cama, Cope, Delcid, Di-Gel, Gacid, Gas Ban DS, Gaviscon, Kudrox, Maalox, Maalox Plus, Mylanta, Mylanta II, Presalin

GENERIC MEDICATION: Aspirin (Acetylsalicylic acid)

BRAND NAMES:

A.S.A., Aspergum, Aspirtab, Asprimox, Bayer, Easprin, Ecotrin, Empirin, GenPrin, Halfprin 81, Heartline, Norwich Aspirin, St. Joseph

ASPIRIN IN COMBINATIONS:

Adprin-B, Alka-Seltzer, Anacin, A.P.C., Arthritis Pain Formula, BC, Ascriptin, Asprimox, Bayer medications, BC Arthritis Strength, Buffaprin, Bufferin, Cama, Cope, Excedrin Extra Strength, Goody's, Midol, Momentum, P-A-C Analgesia, Presalin, Saleto, Sine-Off, Vanquish

GENERIC MEDICATION: Bacitracin

BRAND NAMES:

Baciguent, Bacitracin-Neomycin, Bactine First Aid Antibiotic, Band-Aid Mycitracin, Neosporin Ointment, Polysporin Ointment, Spectro-Biotic, Spectrocin Plus, Tigo, Tri-Biozene, Trimixin, Triple Antibiotic

GENERIC MEDICATION: Benzocaine

BRAND NAMES:

BanSmoke, Cepacol Maximum Strength, SensoGARD, Trocaine

BENZOCAINE IN COMBINATIONS:

Aerotherm, Americaine, Anacaine, Anbesol, Benzo-C, Benzodent, Bicozene, Boil-Ease, Calamatum, Cepacol, Chiggerex, Chigger-Tox, Cough-X, Culminal, Dent's, Dermoplast, Detane, Hurricaine, Jiffy, Lanacane, Medicone, Orabase with Benzocaine, Orajel, Rectal Medicone, Solarcaine, Spec-T Sore Throat, Tanac, Toothache, Zilactin-B

GENERIC MEDICATION: Benzoyl Peroxide

BRAND NAMES:

Acne-5, Acne-10, AMBI, Benoxyl, Clearasil 10%, Clearasil Maximum Strength, Clinac, ExACT, Fostex, Fostex-10%, Oxy-5, Oxy-10 Maximum Strength, Oxy Wash, Panoxyl, Peroxin, Vanoxide

GENERIC MEDICATION: Bisacodyl

BRAND NAMES:

Alophen, Bisac-Evac, Correctol, Dacodyl, Deficol, Delco-Lax, Dulcagen, Dulcolax, Feen-A-Mint, Fleet Laxative, Modane, Reliable Gentle Laxative, Woman's Gentle Laxative

GENERIC MEDICATION: Brompheniramine

BRAND NAMES:

Bromanate, Bromatap, Bromfed, Comtrex Maximum Strength Acute Head Cold Caplets, Dimaphen, Dimetane, Dimetapp, Dristan Allergy, Drixoral Allergy Sinus, Drixoral Cold & Allergy, Drixoral Cold & Flu, Robitussin Allergy & Cough

GENERIC MEDICATION: Caffeine

BRAND NAMES:

Caffedrine, Enerjets, Fastiene, Keep Alert, Keep Going, Molie, No Doz, Overtime, Stay Alert, Stay Awake, 357 HR Magnum, 20-20, Valentine, Vivarin

CAFFEINE IN COMBINATIONS:

Alka-Seltzer Morning Relief, Anacin, APAP-Plus, BC Arthritis Strength, Cope, Excedrin Aspirin-Free, Excedrin Extra Strength, Fendol, Goody's, Saleto, Summit Extra Strength, Vanquish

GENERIC MEDICATION: Calamine

BRAND NAMES:

Aveeno Anti-Itch, Caladryl, Calahist, Calamatum, Calamox, Calamycin, Ivarest, Resinol, Rhuli Spray

GENERIC MEDICATION: Calcium

BRAND NAMES:

Cal-Carb Forte, Calci-Chew, Calci-Mix, Cal-Citrate, Calcium 600, Cal-Lac, Caltrate 600, Citracal, Florical, Nephro-Calci, Os-Cal, Oyst-Cal 500, Posture, Tums.

GENERIC MEDICATION: Calcium Carbonate and Calcium Carbimide

BRAND NAMES:

Alka-Mints, Amitone, Antacid, Cal-Carb Forte, Chooz, Dicarbosil, Maalox, Mallamint, Mylanta, Rolaids, Surpass, Tums

CALCIUM CARBONATE IN COMBINATIONS:

Acid-X, Alkets, Magnebind-200, Mylanta, Natabec, Pepcid Complete, Titralac

GENERIC MEDICATION: Camphor
BRAND NAMES:

Anbesol, Arthricare Double Ice, Aveeno Anti-Itch, Banalg, Blue Star, Caladryl, Campho-Phenique, Chiggerex, Deep-Down, Dencorub, Heet, Mentholatum, Minit-Rub, Noxema Medicated Skin Cream, Rhuli, Sarna, Soltice Quick Rub, Sports Spray Extra Strength, TheraPatch, Vicks Cough Drops, Vicks VapoRub, Vicks VapoSteam

GENERIC MEDICATION: Capsaicin
BRAND NAMES:

Capsin, Capzasin-P, Dolorac, Heet, No Pain-HP, Pain Doctor, Pain-X, R-Gel, Rid-A-Pain, Sloan's, Zostrix

GENERIC MEDICATION: Casanthranol
BRAND NAMES:

Calotabs, Dialose Plus, Dio-Soft, Doxidan, DSS 100 Plus, Easy-Lax, Genasoft Plus, Peri-Colace, Peri-Dos, Pro-Sof, Silace-C

GENERIC MEDICATION: Chlorpheniramine
BRAND NAMES:

Allergy, Chlo-Amine, Chloren, Chlor-Span, Chlor-Trimeton Allergy, Effidac 24, Histacon, Teldrin

CHLORPHENIRAMINE IN COMBINATIONS:

Actifed Cold & Sinus, Al-Ay, Alka-Seltzer Plus Cold, Allerest Maximum Strength, Allergy, BC Allergy Plus, Cerose, CoApap, Cold-Gest, Comtrex Maximum Strength Flu Therapy, Coricidin HBP Cold & Flu, Cotylenol Cold Formula, Decodult, Decohistine,

Dristan Cold & Flu, Drucon, Dryphen, Father John's Medicine Plus, F.C.A.H. Genacol, Gendecon, Good Sense, Hayfebrol, Histatab Plus, Histine 4,8,12, Kolephrin, Mapap CF, PediaCare Night Rest Cough-Cold Formula, Rescon-DM, Robitussin Flu, Robitussin Honey Flu Nighttime, Ryna, Scot-Tossin DM, Sinarest Extra Strength, Sinarest Sinus, Sine-Off Sinus, Singlet, Sinutab Sinus Allergy Medication Maximum Strength, Sudafed Sinus & Allergy, TheraFlu Cold & Cough Nighttime, Thera-Hist Cold & Allergy, Top Care Multi-Symptom Pain Relief Cold, Triacting Cold & Allergy, Triaminic Cold & Allergy, Triaminic Cold & Cough, Tricodene Sugar Free, Tylenol Allergy Sinus Maximum Strength, Vicks 44M Cough and Cold Relief

GENERIC MEDICATION: Coal Tar

BRAND NAMES:

Balnetar, Creamy Tar, Denorex, Doak Tar, Doktar, Estar, High Potency Tar, Ionil T, Lavatar, L.C.D., MG 217, Pentrax, Pentrax Gold, Polytar, Psorigel, PsoriNail, Tarpaste, Tegrin Dandruff Shampoo, Zetar

GENERIC MEDICATION: Dextromethorphan (DM)

BRAND NAMES:

Benylin, Delsym, DexAlone, Mediquell, Scot-Tussin DM, Silphen DM, St. Joseph Cough, Sucrets 4-Hour Cough

DEXTROMETHORPHAN IN COMBINATIONS:

Alka-Seltzer Plus Cough and Cold, Alka-Seltzer Plus Flu, Alka-Seltzer Plus Night-Time Cold Medicine, All-Nite Cold Formula, Ambenyl D, Anti-Tuss DM, Benylin Adult Cough Formula, Benylin DM, Cerose, Cheracol D, Cheracol Plus, Clear Cough DM, Clear Tussin 30, CoApap, Codimal DM, Comtrex Maximum Strength Cold & Cough, Contac Severe Cold and Flu Maximum Strength, Coricidin HBP Cough and Cold, CoTylenol Cold Formula, Cough-X, Delsym, Diabetic Tussin, Diabetic Tussin DM, Diabetic Tussin Maximum Strength, Dimacol, Dimetapp Cold and Cough Maximum Strength, Dimetapp DM, DM Cough, Dristan Cold and

Flu, Drixoral Cough and Congestion Caps, Drixoral Cough Liquid Caps, Drixoral Sore Throat Liquid Caps, Father John's Medicine Plus, Genatuss DM, Genite, Guiatuss CF, Hold, Kolephrin GG/DM, Naldecon DX, Nighttime Cold/Flu, Nite Time Cold Formula, Novahistine DMX, PediaCare Cough & Cold Formula, PediaCare Night Rest Cough-Cold Formula, Pertussin, Pinex, REM, Robafen CF, Robitussin Allergy & Cough, Robitussin CF, Robitussin Cough Drops, Robitussin Honey Cough, Robitussin Maximum Strength Cough, Robitussin Maximum Strength Cough and Cold, Safe Tussin, Scot-Tussin DM, Scot-Tussin Senior, Spec-T Sore Throat Cough Suppressant, St. Joseph Cough Suppressant, Sucrets 4-Hour Cough Suppressant, Sudafed Cold and Cough, Sudafed Severe Cold, TheraFlu Maximum Strength Flu & Cough Night-Time, Triaminic Cold & Cough, Tricodene Sugar Free, Tylenol Cold Multi-Symptom Formula, Tylenol Flu Maximum Strength, Vicks 44 Cough Relief, Vicks 44D Cough and Head Congestion Relief, Vicks 44D Soothing Cough and Head Congestion Relief, Vicks 44E Cough and Chest Congestion Relief, Vicks 44M Pediatric Cough and Cold Relief, Vicks 44M Soothing, Cough, Cold and Flu Relief, Vicks DayQuil LiquiCaps Multi-Symptom Cold/Flu Relief, Vicks NyQuil Cough

GENERIC MEDICATION: Dimenhydrinate
BRAND NAMES:
   Dimenest, Dimentabs, Dinate, Dramamine, Dramanate, Dymenate, Hydrate, Signate, Traveltabs, Triptone, Vertab, VitaHist Oral Spray

GENERIC MEDICATIONS:Diphenhydramine
BRAND NAMES:
   AllerMax, Banophen, Benadryl, Benylin Cough, Dermamycin, Dermarest, Diphen, Diphenhist, Fenylhist, Genahist, Histine 25, Histine 50, Scot-Tussin Allergy, Siladryl, Silphen Cough, Simply Sleep, Sominex, Snooze Fast, Unisom with Pain Relief

DIPHENHYDRAMINE IN COMBINATIONS:

Actifed Allergy Nighttime, Actifed Sinus Nighttime, Alka-Seltzer PM, Banophen Allergy, Bayer PM, Benadryl medications, Compoz, Excedrin PM, Ivarest Maximum Strength, Legatrin PM, Midol PM, Nervene Nighttime, Nytol, Scot-Tussin Allergy Relief, Sleep-EZE, Tylenol Flu Nighttime Maximum Strength Hot Medication, Tylenol PM, Tylenol Severe Allergy, Unisom Pain Relief

GENERIC MEDICATION: Docusate Salts
BRAND NAMES:

Colace, Correctol Extra Gentle, DC Softgels, Dioctolose, Diosate, Docu, D.O.S., Doss, Doxidan, D-S-S, Duosol, Easy-Lax, ex-lax Stool Softener, Genasoft, Konsto, Modane Soft, Peri-Dos, Phillips' Laxcaps, Phillips' Liquigels, Regulax SS, Silace, Stulex, Surfak

DOCUSATE SALTS IN COMBINATIONS:

Calotabs, Dio-Soft, Doxidan, DSS 100 Plus, Easy Lax, ex-lax Gentle Strength, Genasoft Plus, Peri-Colace, Senokot S

GENERIC MEDICATION: Doxylamine
BRAND NAMES:

Alka-Seltzer Plus Night-Time Cold Medicine, All-Nite Cold Formula , Decapryn, Genite, Top Care LiquiCaps Nite Time Multi-Symptom Cold/Flu Relief, Tylenol Sinus Maximum Strenght Nighttime, Unisom Nighttime Sleep Aid, Vicks NyQuil Cough, Vicks NyQuil Liquicaps

GENERIC MEDICATION: Guaifenesin (C)
BRAND NAMES:

Anti-Tuss, Benylin Expectorant, Diabetic Tussin, Glycotuss, Glytuss, G-100, Guiatuss, Humibid, Hytuss, Robitussin, Scot-Tussin Expectorant, Siltussin, Tusibron

GUAIFENESIN IN COMBINATIONS:

Ambenyl-D, Anatuss DM, Anti-Tuss DM, Aspirin-Free Bayer Select Head & Chest Cold, Benylin Multi-Symptom, Brexin-EX, Bronkaid Dual Action, Cheracol Cough, Cheracol D, Clear Cough DM, Clear Tussin 30, Comtrex Multi-Symptom Deep Chest Cold, Congestac, Coricidin Children's Cough, Dexafed, Diabetes CF, Diabetic Tussin DM, Diabetic Tussin EX, Diabetic Tussin Maximum Strength, Dimacol, Dimetane, Dynafed Asthma Relief, Extra Action Cough, Genatuss DM, Glycofed, Glycotuss-DM, Guaifed, Guaifenesin DM, Guaitab, Guiatuss CF, Guiatuss PE, Guistrey Fortis, Kolephrin GG/DM, Mini Two-Way Action, Mytussin, Naldecon Senior DX, Novahistine DMX, Phanatuss, Primatene, Refenesen Plus, Robafen CF, Robafen PE, Robitussin CF, DM, PE, Safe Tussin, Scotcof, Scot-Tussin Senior Clear, Siltussin DM, Sinutab Non-Drying, Sorbase Cough, Sudafed Cold & Cough, Synacol CF, TheraFlu Maximum Strength Flu & Congestion, Tolu-Sed, Triacting, Triaminic Chest Congestion, Triaminic Expectorant, Tusibron, Tussex Cough, Tylenol Cold Multi-Symptom Severe Congestion, Vicks Cough & Chest Congestion Relief, Wal-Tussin DM

GENERIC MEDICATION: Hydrocortisone

BRAND NAMES:

Alphaderm, Anusol-HC, Bactine Hydrocortisone, CaldeCORT, Cortaid, Coticaine Maximum Strength, Cortizone-5, Cortizone-10, Delacort, Dermarest, Dermolate, FoilleCort, HC-DermaPax, Hydroskin, Lanacort, Procort, T/Scalp

HYDROCORTISONE IN COMBINATIONS:

Hysone, Preparation H, Rectal Medicone, Wyanoids HC

GENERIC MEDICATION: Ibuprofen

BRAND NAMES:

Advil medications, Dristan Sinus, Excedrin IB, Genpril, Haltran, Menadol, Midol IB, Midol Maximum Strength, Motrin IB, Nuprin, Saleto 200, Sine-Aid IB

GENERIC MEDICATION: Iron

BRAND NAMES:

Childron, C-Ron, Cytoferrin,Eldofe, El-Ped-Ron, Farbegen, Feco-T, Femiron, Feosol, Feostat, Ferancee, Feratab, Fer-gen-sol, Fergon, Fer-In-Sol, Fer-Iron, Fero-Folic 500, Fero-Grad-500, Fero-Gradumet, Ferolix, Fer-Regules, Ferretts, Ferro-Docusate TR, Ferro-Dok, Ferro-DSS SR, Ferrodyl, Ferromar, Ferro-Sequels, Fesotyme, Folvron, Fumasorb, Fumerin, Hemocyte, Irospan, Ircon, Laud-Iron, Maniron, Min-Hema, Mol-Iron, Nephro-Fer, Slow Fe, Stuart Hematinic

GENERIC MEDICATION: Kaolin

BRAND NAMES:

B-K-P, Diastop, Kaodene Non-Narcotic, Kaopectate, Kaospen, Kao-Tin, Kapectin, Pecto-Kalin

GENERIC MEDICATION: Magnesium Salts

BRAND NAMES:

Almora, Alsorb, Aludrox, Arcodex, Ascriptin, Banacid, Cope, Delcid, Di-Gel, Gacid, Gas Ban DS, Gaviscon, Haley's M-O, Maalox, Mag-G, Magonate, Magtrate, Maracid 2, Medalox Gel, Mylanta, Pepcid Complete, Phillips' Milk Of Magnesia, Riopan, Rolaids

GENERIC MEDICATION: Menthol

BRAND NAMES:

AllerMax Allergy & Cough Formula, BenGay, Blue Gel Muscular Pain Reliever, Cepacol, Deep Down, Dencorub, Dermoplast Spray, Diabetic Tussin Cough Drops, Diabetic Tussin EX, Diphen Cough, Eucalyptamint Maximum Strength, Guaifed Syrup, Halls Cough Drops, Isodettes, Luden's Cough Drops, Mentholatum, N'Ice, Robitussin Honey Calmers, Robitussin Honey Cough Drops, Scot-Tussin Expectorant, Sucrets 4-Hour Cough,Thera-Gesic Crème, Tricodene Sugar Free, Vicks Cough Drops, Vicks Vaporub, Victor's

GENERIC MEDICATION: Miconazole

BRAND NAMES:

Breezee-Mist Antifungal, Desenex Antifungal, Desenex Cream, Fungoid Tincture, Micatin, Monistat, Ting, Zeasorb-AF

GENERIC MEDICATION: Naphazoline

BRAND NAMES:

All Clear, Allerest Eye Drops, Clear Eyes, Comfort Eye Drops, Degest-2, Muro's Opcon, Naphcon A, Privine, VasoClear, Vasocon, Visine A Eye Drops

GENERIC MEDICATION: Neomycin

BRAND NAMES:

Lanabiotic, Myciguent, Mycitracin, Neosporin, Spectrocin Plus, Tigo, Trimixin, Triple Antibiotic

GENERIC MEDICATION: Oxymetazoline Hydrochloride

BRAND NAMES:

Afrin Nasal Spray, Allerest Nasal Spray, Chlorphed-LA, Dristan 12-Hour Nasal Spray, Duramist Plus 12-Hour Decongestant, Duration, Neosynephrine Nasal Spray, Nostrilla 12-Hour, NTZ, Sinarest Decongestant, Twice-A-Day 12-Hour Nasal, Vicks Sinex 12-Hour Nasal Spray, Visine L.R. Eye Drops

GENERIC MEDICATION: Phenylephrine

BRAND NAMES:

Acotus, Alcon-Efrin, Alka-Seltzer Plus Cold & Cough Medicine, Alka-Seltzer Plus Cold, Alka-Seltzer Plus Night-Time Cold Medicine, Cerose, Codimal DM, Decodult, Dexafed, Dimetane, Doktor's Spray, Dondril, Dristan Nasal Mist, Dryphen Multi-Symptom Formula, Ephrine Nasal Spray, Father John's Medicine Plus, Fendol, Formulation R, Gendecon, Histatab-Plus, Hista-Vent DA, Neo-Synephrine, Omnicol, Prefrin, Preparation H, Rescon-

GG, Relief, Rhinall, Sinarest, Tussex Cough, Vicks Sinex Nasal Spray

GENERIC MEDICATION: Polymixin b
BRAND NAMES:
Band Aid Plus, Betadine First Aid Antibiotics, Double Antibiotic, Lanabiotic, Mycitracin, Neosporin, Polysporin, Spectrocin Plus, Tigo, Tri-Biozene, Trimixin, Triple Antibiotic

GENERIC MEDICATION: Pramoxine Hydrochloride
BRAND NAMES:
Anti-Itch, Anusol Ointment, Aveeno Anti-Itch, Caladryl, Calamycin, Fleet Pain-Relief, Hemorid for Women, Itch-X, Pramegel, Prax, Procto Foam, Tronolane Cream

GENERIC MEDICATION: Pseudoephedrine
BRAND NAMES:
Actifed Cold & Allergy, Actifed Cold & Sinus, Advil Flu & Body Ache, Allerest Maximum Strength, Aleve Cold & Sinus, Aleve Sinus & Headache, Alka-Seltzer Plus Cold, Alka-Seltzer Plus Night-Time Cold Liqui-gels, All-Nite Cold Formula, Ambenyl-D, BC Allergy Sinus Cold Powder, BC Sinus Cold Powder, Benadryl Allergy & Cold, Benadryl Allergy & Sinus, Benadryl Allergy & Sinus Headache, Benadryl Maximum Strength Severe Allergy & Sinus Headache, Benylin Multi-Symptom, Brexin, Bromfed, Chlor-Trimeton Allergy-D, Co-Apap, Codimal, Comtrex medications, Congestac, Contac medications, Coricidin D Cold Flu & Sinus, CoTylenol Cold Formula, Dimacol Dimetane, Dimetapp DM Cold & Cough, Dimetapp Nighttime Flu, Dimetapp Non-Drowsy Flu, Dorcol Children's Cough, Dristan Cold, Dristan Sinus, Drixoral Allergy Sinus, Drixoral Cold & Allergy, Drixoral Cold & Flu, Excedrin Sinus, Genite, Glycofed, Good Sense Maximum Strength Dose Sinus, Good Sense Maximum Strength Pain Relief Allergy, Guaifed, Guaitab, Guiatuss, Guiatuss CF, Hayfebrol,

Kolephrin/DM Caplets, Mapap Cold Formula, Motrin Children's Cold Oral Suspension, Motrin Sinus/Headache, Novahistine DMX, Nytcold Medicine, Nytime Cold Medicine, Ornex No Drowsiness, PediaCare medications, Pertussin All Night PM, Primatuss Cough Mixture 4D, Robitussin Allergy & Cough, Robitussin Cold Cold & Congestion, Robitussin Cold Multi-Symptom Cold & Flu, Robitussin CF, Robitussin Flu, Robitussin Honey Flu Nighttime, Robitussin Maximum Strength Cough & Cold, Robitussin Multi-Symptom Honey Flu, Robitussin PE, Robitussin Sinus & Congestion, Rhinosyn, Scot-Tussin Hayfebrol, Sine-Off, Singlet, Sinutab Sinus Allergy Medication Maximum Strength Formula, Sinutab Sinus Medication Maximum Strength Without Drowsiness Formula, Sudafed medications, Tavist Allergy/Sinus/Headache, TheraFlu medications, Top Care Maximum Strength Flu Cold & Cough Medicine Night Time, Top Care Multi-Symptom Pain Relief Cold, Triaminic medications, Ty-Cold, Tylenol Allergy Sinus, Tylenol Maximum Strength Allergy Sinus NightTime, Tylenol Cold Multi-Symptom Severe Congestion, Tylenol Flu Maximum Strength Nighttime, Tylenol Flu Maximum Strength Non-Drowsy, Tylenol Maximum Strength Nighttime, Tylenol Sinus, Vicks 44D Cough & Head Congestion Relief, Vicks 44M Cough Cold & Flu Relief, Vicks DayQuil LiquiCaps Multi-Symptom Cold/Flu Relief

GENERIC MEDICATION: Psyllium
BRAND NAMES:

Fiberall, Gen Fiber; Hydrocil Instant, Konsyl, Metamucil, Modane Bulk, Natural Fiber, Perdiem, Reguloid, Serutan, StePhan Relief Capsules, Syllact

GENERIC MEDICATION: Resorcinol
BRAND NAMES:

Acnomel, Acnotex, Bicozene, Black and White Ointment, Clearasil Adult Care Cream, Lanacane, Resinol, Rezamid, Vagisil

GENERIC MEDICATION: Salicylates

BRAND NAMES:

Anodynos, Backache, Cystex, Deep Down, Dencorub, Doan's Pills, Heet, Mobigesic, Momentum

GENERIC MEDICATION: Salicylic Acid

BRAND NAMES:

Acno, AMBI 10, Aveenobar Medicated, Clean and Clear Invisible Blemish Treatment, Clean and Clear Oil Controlling Astringent, Clear Away One-Step Wart Remover, Clear Away Plantar Wart Remover, Clearasil Clearstick, Compound W, Corn Fix, Doctor Scholl's, Drytex, DulFilm Liquid Wart Remover, DuoPlant Plantar Wart Remover, ExACT Pore Treatment, Fostex Medicated, Fung-O, Gordofilm, Mosco Corn and Callus Remover, Neutrogena Clear Pore Treatment, Occlusal HP, OFF-Ezy Products, Oxy Deep Cleansing, Oxy Night Watch Maximum Strength, Pernox, Propa pH Acne Medicines, Sal-Acid Wart Remover, SalAc Cleanser, Salactic Film, Sal-Plant, Sebasorb, Stri-Dex Products, Therac, Trans-Ver-Sal, Wart Off

GENERIC MEDICATION: Senna and Sennocides

BRAND NAMES:

Agoral, Dosaflex, ex-lax, Fletcher's Castoria, Gentle Nature, Nature's Remedy, Perdiem, Senexon, Senna-Gen, Senokot

GENERIC MEDICATION: Simethicone (C)

BRAND NAMES:

Anti-Gas, Di-Gel, Gas Ban, Gas Relief, Gas-X, Genasyme, Kudrox, Losopan Plus, Maalox Antacid/Anti-Gas, Maalox Plus, Mylanta II, Mylicon, Phazyme, Riopan Plus, Tempo, Titralac Plus, Tums Plus

GENERIC MEDICATION: Sulphur

BRAND NAMES:

Acno, Acnomel, Acnotex, Bensulfoid, Clearasil Adult Care Cream, Fostex, Fostril, Meted, Pernox, Poslam Psoriasis, Rezamid, SAStid, Sebulex, Sulfoam, Sulforcin, Sulmasque, Sulpho-Lac, Sulray, Therac, Thylox Acne

GENERIC MEDICATION: Tolnaftate

BRAND NAMES:

Absorbine Jr. Antifungal, Blis-To-Sol (Liquid), Dr. Scholl's, Genaspor, Johnson's Odor-Eaters, NP-27, Tinactin

GENERIC MEDICATION: Triprolidine

BRAND NAMES:

Actifed Cold & Allergy, Allerfrim, Aprodine, Cenafed Plus, Genac, Silafed, Sudafed Sinus Nighttime

GENERIC MEDICATION: Zinc Oxide

BRAND NAMES:

Ammens, Anusol, Anusol HC, Balmex, Calamycin, Caldesene Medicated Ointment, Desitin, Diaperene Diaper Rash, Diaper Guard, Diaper Rash Ointment, Dyprotex, Flanders Buttocks, Fostril, Hem-Prep, Little Bottoms, Mexsana Medicated, Ostiderm, Pazo, Plexolan Lanolin, Resinol, Schamberg's Anti-Itch, Wyanoids